THE ROAD LESS TAKEN

LESSONS FROM A LIFE SPENT CYCLING

KATHRYN BERTINE

TRIUMPH
BOOKS ®

TRIUMPHBOOKS**.COM**

This book is available in quantity at special discounts for your group or organization. For further information, contact:

Triumph Books LLC
814 North Franklin Street
Chicago, Illinois 60610
(312) 337-0747
Fax (312) 280-5470
www.triumphbooks.com

Printed in U.S.A.

ISBN: 978-1-62937-012-5

Design by Amy Carter

All photos courtesy of the author unless otherwise indicated.

TO MY SISTERHOOD OF PRO CYCLING.
YOU CHOSE THE RIGHT ROAD.

*"I WENT ON A SEARCH FOR SOMETHING REAL,
TRADED WHAT I KNOW FOR HOW I FEEL."*

—The Avett Brothers

*"WHEN THE GOING GETS WEIRD, THE WEIRD
TURN PRO."*

—Hunter S. Thompson

CONTENTS

FOREWORD

by Lindsay Berra, national correspondent for MLB.com

I WAS A 19-YEAR-OLD college sophomore, home from Christmas break in 1996. I got a package in the mail from Amazon.com. Inside, I found a copy of Stephen Ambrose's book, *Undaunted Courage*, about the Lewis and Clark expedition to unlock the American West. The note inside from Dr. John J. McMullen said, "I thought you would like this."

First, let's acknowledge that the Internet was still little more than a precocious toddler in 1996, and that Dr. Mac, who was nearly 80 at the time, had already figured it out. He was always a pioneer of sorts. He was a retired naval commander who ran a very successful shipping business, but he loved sports, too. He brought the National Hockey League's New Jersey Devils into a market already saturated with New York Rangers fans—where no one believed a team could thrive, much less win—and went on to collect three Stanley Cups. And as the owner of baseball's Houston Astros, he hired Bob Watson as the GM. Watson was just the second African American to hold that position in Major League Baseball.

Dr. Mac was also the reason I met Kate Bertine.

Yes, I've known Kathryn long enough that I still call her Kate. Calling her by her childhood nickname is a habit I've been unable to get my tongue to break. To me, Kate is still the same teenager I met at the Meadowlands in the

'90s, all wide-eyes, long legs, and bangs. But she likes to use her Big-Girl Name, so henceforth, I will use it, too.

Both Kathryn's parents and my grandparents were lucky enough to call Dr. Mac a friend, and we would all meet at Brendan Byrne Arena to watch the Devils play. Kathryn and I would eat chicken fingers and lean through the windows of Suite 121, transfixed by the action on the ice below. Dr. Mac always got a kick out of us—two girls who knew the intricacies of line changes and the two-line pass better than any of the men in the room. And because he was such a smart fellow, I think Dr. Mac knew Kathryn and I would be holding our own with the men for the rest of our lives.

By that time, I was already playing high school hockey. Boys hockey, that is; my high school didn't have a girls team, and by my senior year, I was captain of the varsity team. My high school team practiced and played at the same rink in suburban New Jersey where the Devils practiced, and sometimes, I'd hop the boards after a shift and see my grandfather and Dr. Mac, eyeing me up from the other side of the glass. They were tough to impress and would never clap or cheer or shout. The best I would get was a nod of approval after a sneaky back-door goal or a tough battle along the half-wall against a boy twice my size. I know they both thought I was a little nuts, but I also know they appreciated my kind of crazy. Kathryn's kind of crazy.

Dr. Mac and I got along. He approved of my gumption, encouraged my wanderlust, and seemed to understand them both more than either of my parents. He always stayed on top of what I was up to. I went to college at the University of North Carolina at Chapel Hill, where I continued to play hockey on the men's club team. I also walked on to the varsity softball team, which was a considerable accomplishment for an unrecruited player from the Northeast. After college, I became a writer for *ESPN The Magazine*, where I traveled more than 200 days a year both nationally and internationally for better than a decade, covering hockey, tennis, and baseball (my bread-and-butter sports) and other sports, too—everything from boxing and snowboarding to college hoops and roller derby. And always, I was one of the only women in the pressbox, in the lockerroom, on the field. Now, as a national correspondent at MLB.com, the same is true.

I work in much the same way I played—head down, nose-to-the-grindstone, doing the best job I can possibly do. It's the same way Kathryn rides her bike. It's the way we both live our lives.

We both travel, a lot. Sure, a lot of it is work-related, but there are also a lot of trips we choose to take because there's a mountain we want to climb or a beautiful stretch of road we want to ride. I like to think of my sense of adventure as one of my best qualities, but it often leads to that same presumptuous question, one that I know Kathryn also hears, over and over: "Don't you think it's time to settle down?" That query always makes me think of great white sharks and automatic watches; if they stop moving, they'll die.

That question also reminds me of the 592-page thumbs-up I once received from a man who didn't dole out thumbs-ups very liberally. Dr. Mac told me to follow my own path by giving me the story of two men who quite literally made their own.

Kathryn and I have always had that in common—we've done what has made us happy with little regard for what everyone else says should make us happy. I won't apologize for that, and I don't think Kathryn ever will, either.

It's like she says; the wind feels too good on our faces.

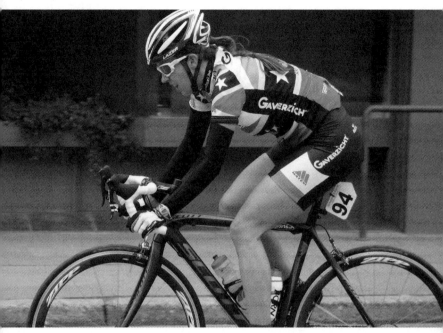

I only look like I know where I am going.

INTRODUCTION

AT 18, I KNEW exactly where my life would be by the time I turned 28. I'd be married, have two kids, maybe three. There would be a medium-sized dog of mixed-breed heritage, pound rescued. My job within the publishing industry would be steady—no, lucrative!—and my income within a comfortable upper-middle-class bracket. So that's what I wrote down in the spring of 1993 when my high school history teacher, Mr. Johnson, handed each student in his senior homeroom a blank sheet of paper and asked where we saw ourselves 10 years later, when the calendar brought forth 2003.

Bil Johnson was the man. The dude. The cool teacher. The one with the ponytail, the hip wardrobe, and a passion for teaching accented with a slight, unspoken disdain for the syllabi and structures that steered students toward test-score prowess instead of an education based on truly absorbing the lessons of the world. His full name was Wilbur. I applauded his savvy commitment to being a Bil with one "l." As a Kathryn called Katie during my childhood, it made no sense that my parents chose "-ie" instead of Katy. Bil Johnson was my hero, a much-needed sign there were people in this world who *got it*. Despite the fact I had no idea what "it" was. This naiveté was clear, as my 10-year prediction of my life mirrored exactly the same sentiments as most of the other girls in my class. We simply used our moms as models for the question, calculating how old they'd been when we were born, where we lived in New York suburbia, and what some of our parents did for a living. I lived in the right town, went to the right school, kept myself in the right lane, and that was that. I'd surely stay in the right lane and keep making right turns.

Bil Johnson collected our letters. He said he'd mail them to us in 10 years. We snickered.

In 2003 my parents received a letter addressed to me. They had moved six years prior from the house I grew up in, but our town was small and my parents had not moved far. The postman remembered the new house and dropped the letter in their new mailbox. I, too, had moved many times since college. My parents forwarded the letter to

Colorado, where I lived in a rented home with three house-mates on the outskirts of Boulder. I was struggling to find work and had recently broken up with a serious boyfriend. I was 28 and batting zero for the very predictions I made about my own life. I had *nothing* my teenage self thought I'd have—no husband, no kids, no dog, no salary. And yet, there was this: I was happy. I liked my life, unpredictable and oblique as it was.

There I stood, holding a letter from the past written about the future mailed by an old history teacher forcing me to contemplate the present. My first reaction was to laugh at everything from my gullibility and sentimental-ity to the fact I'd so assuredly written my future in pencil. As the letter lingered in my thoughts, which was surely what Bil Johnson intended, my feelings turned inward and one question drifted to the forefront. Though I was happy, I was struggling. *Is it okay that I've veered so far off course? To miss the right-turn lane? To have amassed nothing from the realms of my own projected normalcy?* It would take another decade to formally decide on such answers.

Now, at 38, I know the answer to veering from the path of normalcy is yes, it is okay. Not only is it okay to take the road less traveled, but it's the one we're supposed to take if we're lucky enough to see a divergence. I don't think this alternative path shows itself to everyone, and that is also okay. But for those of us who do see it, or want to see it, the road shows up for a reason. Not necessarily a spiritual "reason" as I'm not likening this road to a religious or uni-versal belief, nor can I attest that this reason is a biological impulse. Reason itself may be none or all of those things, but I do believe we're all born with an internal What-If whisper. Some of us just hear it louder than others. For this reason, I've never thought that Robert Frost actually *chose* between the two roads in his famous poem, "The Road Not Taken." Sure, he saw two roads and looked at them both. He admits they were both pretty equal. Then he took one. Yet in using the word "take" instead of "choose," I've always felt as if Frost possessed that What-If whisper, the one that says, "Come on, Bob. This really isn't a choice. You know you're supposed to take that path on the left. So get on it."[1]

My whispers, paths, and What-Ifs led me far from the predictions of an 18-year-old girl who had yet to understand the gorgeous, gnarled maps of Maybe that would soon unfurl their atlas within me.

As a child, I fell in love with sports. Only as any athlete knows, sport itself isn't so much the draw as the energy, will, and passion it brings out within us. In high school I ran cross country because I was drawn to the hunt of chasing down my competition, and I came to respect this primordial lesson of persistence. In college I rowed, engulfed by the physical understanding of harmony and unison and balance, and how life seemed most perfect when surrounded by those who also treasured such measurements of joy. After college, I took a road most definitely less traveled and signed on for a year of professional figure skating with companies like Ice Capades, Holiday on Ice, and Hollywood on Ice. Skating was my first true love, a

---

[1] Frost's famous poem draws countless debate from literary critics. While many readers find the symbolism of Frost's choices and paths to operate on a level of soulful depth and introspection, others argue the writer's intent was mimicry and sarcasm. Really, can one choice ever be superior to another? Does it even matter what path you take? When asked about "The Road Not Taken," Frost replied, "You have to be careful of that one; it's a tricky poem—very tricky." Well fine, then. So be it. I'll take the trick on the right.

sport that above all else taught me the greatest lesson sport can teach: how to be yourself. Skating was, at its most basic element, a literal exercise in carving one's own path. Yet on the professional tour, I got lost. The path became unclear, my life map suddenly blurred by warring territories where hopes and dreams fought desperately to cross into the borders of reality. What was once a dream to skate with the best disintegrated into the veracity of a second-rate tour of former athletes who had little respect for their bodies, or much else. I struggled then, as the epicenter of an athlete's code—to never give up—clashed terribly with the idea that it's okay to look for a new path when the one we're on becomes a dead end. Years removed from the skating tour, I never regret the decision to take that road. It was a road as right as it was wrong, for any journey that unhinges the control panel of our soul and lets us take a hard look at our own wiring is ultimately a worthwhile quest.[2]

I found the right path after my skating tour, which took me to graduate school in Tucson, Arizona. Without skating, I heeded my body's call to find a new sport and joined the world of triathlon. The swimming, biking, and running dug their hooks into me, and I worked all the odd jobs that allowed me to put sport and writing first. I stayed on the triathlon road for nine years, traveling past my 30th birthday, winding around a couple of tumultuous relationships into the professional realms of racing and publishing my first memoir, *All the Sundays Yet to Come*, moving myself from Tucson to Boulder to the East Coast and back to Tucson again, stumbling off path a few times but somehow knowing that

---

[2] *All The Sundays Yet to Come: A Skater's Journey* gives the full story of the skating tour, published by Little, Brown in 2003.

the stumbles were supposed to be part of the trip. When it comes to the road less traveled, "stumble" is code for "lesson." Of course, some lessons don't always feel so great during the learning process. There were many times where, in the midst of a life lesson, I wanted nothing more than to cut class. Then in the clamorous core of one rather large life tutorial, I stumbled upon a most unbelievable path.

During my freelance career, which somewhat sustained me through the paltry and often nonexistent paychecks of women's professional sports, I'd done a fair bit of work for *ESPN The Magazine*. In 2006, the company approached me to write an online column called "So You Wanna Be an Olympian?" about what it actually takes to get to the modern day Olympic Games. The 2008 Beijing Summer Games were just two years away, and my job was to do whatever it took to qualify. In any sport possible. (I tried a handful of fascinating sports and eventually chose to pursue road cycling.) The ESPN call came at the most interesting time, as I was reeling from my broken engagement to Mr. Wrong Path. At the time, my chosen road was jagged and wobbly and felt as if I were trying to traverse the Himalayas in flip flops. Unexpectedly, ESPN parachuted in and pointed the way. For two and a half years, I embarked on the most incredible, life-altering journey that merged my two passions of sport and writing. *As Good As Gold* was published, chronicling the adventure.

And then, as all things do in the world of publishing and contracted assignments, my road ended. The 2008 Olympics came and went, the book hit the shelves in 2010, the column was finished, and that should have been that in regard to my cycling adventure. Yet something uncharacteristic happened during that Olympic journey. I completely forgot to turn right. Or left. I ended up in the bike lane, kept going straight, and fell deeply in love with road cycling. We began a serious relationship. Every lesson I ever learned in skating, rowing, running, and triathlon found the ultimate classroom in cycling. I was 33 years old in 2008 when the new What-If whispered, "What if you could ride all the way to the professional ranks?"

I knew exactly what I was up against, physically and emotionally. Roads less taken are terrific in many regards but hardly synonymous with continuity or ease. I learned that struggle most often arrives under two circumstances: when we can't see our path, or when we choose to stray from the one we're truly meant to follow. No path is clear the whole time; there is rarely smooth pavement along the road less traveled. That would be a given. This new goal of cycling toward the pro ranks would bring victory and devastation, difficulty and enlightenment, and yet another detour from the predictions of a life most traveled. I thought of Bil Johnson and how my high school letter of life prediction would probably never come true at this rate, but there on the scroll of old memories and new hopes running through my mind, I was sure I could see him smiling in approval. When the What-If first breathed the idea of racing professionally into me, I knew the goal had little to do with cycling and everything to do with trying. Trying was—and is—my true north, regardless of destination. It has taken 20 years for this realization to surface and solidify. But I now know I am supposed to live a life of peaks and valleys, and while I often yearn for the ease of flatter ground, I am happiest while climbing.

I also understood that this professional cycling goal wasn't a journey of sport but a further expedition of a life less ordinary. One that would chronicle five years of my mid-thirties, no less. Who, at 33, chooses bicycles over babies? Highways over husbands? Carbon fiber over fortuitous careers? No one, surely. That is, no one *chooses*. It is simply who we are to heed our What-Ifs. And the call of the What-If is hardly specific to athletes.

As a writer, it is my belief that sport is just a metaphor no different than any other literary conceit, from mystery and fantasy to love and war. Corporate publishing would disagree. The idea of life lessons learned by a woman on a bicycle means such a book will probably end up on the sports shelf, smushed in with the heroes and how-tos of athleticism, though I wrote it not for athletes but for anyone who has ever had the simplest desire to try something different in their own life. I wrote it for that guy in the cubicle who keeps checking out that webpage about volunteering in Africa. For the waitress wondering about med school. For the mom with three kids who hears that whisper of starting her own company. For the senior citizen tired of the same old, same old, and curious about the brand new, brand new. For the teenager who knows exactly where she'll be in 10 years, and for the 48-year-old who's still searching. And of course, I wrote this for the Bil Johnsons of the world, who send mirrors masked as letters and use words to help us take a look at ourselves.

I may have used a bicycle to find my road less taken, but it was merely the vehicle for a voyage rather than the voyage itself. Most of these pages are about life off the bicycle—all the things I learned while answering the What-Ifs, while I went to find my path. For months, I wracked brains, books, and essays for a scholarly close to this introduction. Surely Plato or Wordsworth or Emerson or Dickens could best express what I wanted to emote, give that one final nugget of guidance and truth about heeding What-Ifs and mustering the tenacity to seek one's true path. Instead, I found my closing inspiration in the most unlikely source—an old Pee-wee Herman movie being broadcast on a third-rate cable network that I surfed past while eating lunch after a long winter-training ride. Just before Pee-wee sets out for his Big Adventure in the silliest of his '80s movies, Herman proclaims with simplistic resolve:

"I'm going to find my bike."

Eventually, he does. May you find yours.

—K.B.

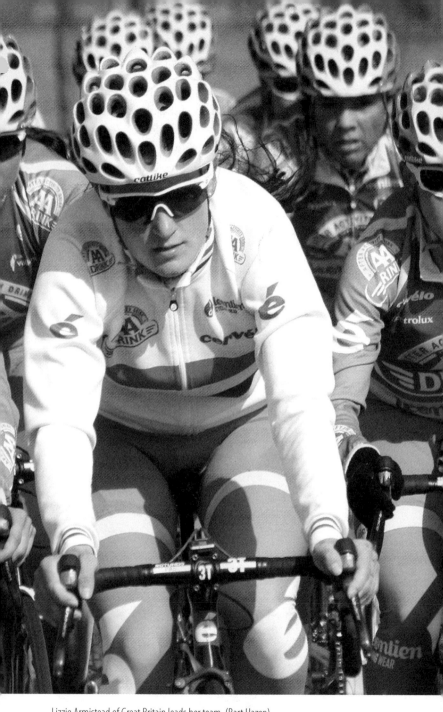

Lizzie Armistead of Great Britain leads her team. (Bart Hazen)

PART I:
SHARE THE ROAD

We are taught from a young age that the gift of sport is a lifelong exercise in perseverance and striving. Traveling around the world, racing my bike, I soon realized the subtle undertones of tolerance were also one of sport's greatest lessons. Whether between rival competitors, the progression of equality, or compassion for fallen heroes, to share the proverbial road is one of cycling's quiet yet most powerful attributes.

THE EMPRESS OF MAYBE
May 2012

MORIAH ATTACKS FIRST. She launches from the left side of the road, her momentum clean, confident, and steady. As she comes around the international peloton of cyclists, a Brazilian rider jumps to go with her. Sprinting away from the bunch, their bicycles rock from side to side with the torque of their frantic effort; two metallic metronomes visually keeping time to a private rhythm of hope and maybe.

Here in San Salvador, the peloton—82 women in total—will pull them back within minutes, its largeness far more efficient than the two cyclists trying to break away from its formation. The peloton is the lion, Moriah the lamb—albeit a lamb who wants to survive. Moriah knows her fate; her daring hustle is part of our strategy. I ready myself for the counter attack. Moving over to the right-hand side of the road, I watch for the deep-set rivets and cracks that run through El Salvador's ancient pavement where bony fingers of tar-encrusted chip seal reach out for our tires, as if to seek hold of our Olympic dreams. Seven days, eight stages, temperatures in the high 90s—the Vuelta El Salvador is a mighty beast of an endurance event.

The moment Moriah is reeled in by the peloton, I surge. Away from the bunch with frenetic adrenaline, I sprint alone up the road. The lion watches but does not react. Not yet. I

2

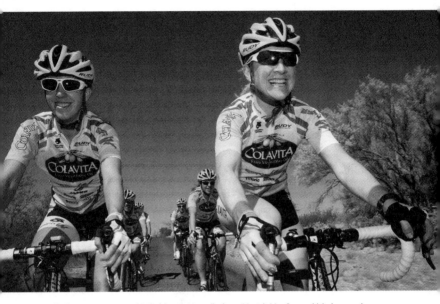

Nothing great is ever achieved (or attempted) alone. Moriah MacGregor (r) helps me chase my Maybes. (Jonathan Devich/epicimages.us)

am simply being stalked, and we both know it. Logic tells me I, too, will be brought back to the peloton, as the 80 women behind me are in no mood to let anyone get away when qualification points for London are on the line. Still, a breakaway is my only hope.

"Only the sprinters will win at the line," Moriah reminds me. "If you want any shot at winning, you need to break way well before the finish. If you go early, they might not chase you."

"Might" is all I need to hear. I have built an emotional empire on might, this strange word that yields definitions of both strength and chance, as if it surreptitiously knows they're the same thing. I used to be paralyzed by Mights and Maybes, unable to see how either could result in anything but should-haves and if-onlys. During the five prior years I spent competing as a bike racer, I grew comfortable at the back of the peloton, reacting to the moves of others instead of initiating my own bouts of chance. I lingered in the realm of "good enough" all the while knowing it wasn't. This attitude would not get me on a professional team, and at 36, there was little time for second chances. For years, coaches and competitors taught me to "push myself," but that term wasn't right for me. I knew exactly how to push and drive and kick and force myself, to physically fight for the elusive next level. The push was ingrained in me. What I needed was the opposite: I needed to understand how to let go. To relish the unknown. To risk blowing up, getting dropped, being left behind, or passed by a lesser athlete. Patience and calmness, these were the lessons that eluded me. I needed to find the strength to be okay with nearly, at one with almost. I had to forget about watts, lactic thresholds, power zones, and intervals and instead train and race toward a new objective: to find strength in chance. To see what happens if I chase down a world champion or attack an Olympian or experiment with emptying my physical and emotional tank before the climb instead of during it. These were the risks that might work, if only I were comfortable with "might." As someone who prefers control, the notion of chance was as frightening as it was foreign. Yet I knew in order to progress, I had to build an empire on might and crown myself the Empress of Maybe. Only then, I finally figured out, could I get where I wanted to go.

I stand on the pedals and dash toward the open sea of pavement. No one comes with me. Moriah is resting in the middle of the lion's belly, protecting herself from wind and exertion as the beast of the peloton breathes its collective breath. I know what the peloton sees up the road is not the Empress of Maybe. They see the white and blue kit of some woman on a local team advertising an El Salvadoran bakery; they see the race number of a rider not on their radar for winning. "Le Croissant," my jersey reads. I am not a threat. I am not even a name. I am, at best, a pastry with gumption. *Let her go*, they think.

Yet a few women in the peloton know my story of trying to make the Beijing Games and assume correctly that I am here again in 2012 to seek enough qualification points to earn a berth to the London Olympics. None have seen me breakaway before, and I feel their eyes on me, assessing my level of potential. It is both a compliment and a curse when a Brazilian domestique—a worker bee for her team's queen—is sent to fetch me. She is the younger cousin of the Fernandes family, a sister-cousin contingent of four riders from Brazil. She sits in my draft, tailing me, not wanting to share the work and help us both get away from the lion but to slow down my pace if I get too far away from the field.

The move is a frustrating one, as the young Brazilian is a strong rider, and perhaps with tandem effort we could escape for a while. But she is working for her cousin, a cyclist just back from a doping suspension. Here, in El Salvador, there is no doping control. While very few of cycling's pro women go down this path of cheating, sometimes in the untested races in faraway locations, the occasional dirty riders mix in with clean ones. But there is no emotional energy or time available to ponder these injustices in the middle of a race. What another rider does to her body is beyond my control. All I can do is use my own and take charge of my Maybes.

The peloton makes its way to the Brazilian and me, and I slide into the middle of the bunch, absorbed into this rolling, shape-shifting amoeba of wheels and lycra. I catch what is left of my breath and watch Moriah jump away once more with three other riders who have siphoned their own private Maybes into the courage to go with her. The peloton tolerates the gap for a few minutes, then slowly hunts them down again.

I ready myself and flee once more into that electrifying chasm between hopeful and hopeless. Catch, release, catch, release, the lion prefers to play with the lamb today rather than make it a meal. The meal will come later. The attack-the-peloton pattern resumes for nearly an hour before my body begins to reel from the physical impact of chasing Maybes. The peloton has overthrown my empire today. I am relegated to second in command, the Empress of Almost. With raspy gasps of emptied effort, I drift down through the middle of the peloton, conscious of little other than the fact this is the end of my day. There is still an hour or so left till the finish, but I will no longer be able to hold onto the peloton. Back, back, I float…passing jerseys from Chile and Venezuela. Back, back…past U.S. and Argentina. Soon I know I'll be adrift and alone, the shores of Antarctica far more likely than London.

Then I feel the hand.

A claw-like grip grabs my right rear jersey pocket, bunching the fabric in what feels like a small fist, and yanks my jersey forward. The movement is sharp and quick, strong yet fleeting. I am being pulled in the opposite direction of my backward momentum. Or am I being pushed? Actually, I'm being flung. I glance left and see who belongs to the hand. My slingshot is Evelyn Garcia, the national champion of El Salvador. She is no more than 5' tall, likely hovering near 100 lbs., yet her small hand on my back may have well been the strength and palm of a mythical giant.

The physical momentum of her fling lasts no more than two seconds, yet within those ephemeral pulses, my legs receive the briefest reprieve…a beat of rest just long enough to renew my soul. It will be this moment—the moment my competition became a teammate and paid her respect to my own private Maybe—that will come to stand as my greatest memory in cycling. Pushing or pulling another human being on a bicycle takes a great deal of energy, strength, and skill, even for a fraction of a moment. To be pushed by a stranger on another team who is also in need of Olympic points gave me something far greater than a few seconds of rest. In the momentary current of that push was something I'd been seeking since I started cycling, a validation that I belonged here among the best. I never quite believed it until that instant. Each athlete has their internal struggles, and doubt has long been mine. Yet this tiny, almost violent flick of momentum whispered not through words but touch, *You belong.* I hang onto the end of the peloton, and finish the day far from first, but neither adrift nor alone. I am not in Antarctica. The lion has not swallowed me. The throne of Maybe sits in wait.

"We'll try again tomorrow," Moriah consoles at the finish line, where we melt into the hot mess of emptied effort and blank thoughts.

"Tomorrow," I exhale.

Moriah pedals off to find our team car, I find a bottle of water and the closest curb. Jerome, one of our team managers, notes the temperature—104 degrees Fahrenheit—and sits near me silently. An athlete himself, he knows this is

7

a time for shade and water, not words and sentiments. I appreciate the silence, which carries on for a good 15 minutes before a gaggle of small children approach timidly and ask for my water bottle.

"*Si, para un foto,*" I bargain with them. Yes, for a photo you can have my water bottle. They gather around and I give the Bloggie, my cheap purple flip camera, to Jerome. He snaps a shot I come to treasure as one of my greatest visual memories of cycling. There are no Olympic points for this, but I can't help but wonder if there should be. There will, in fact, be no points at all for me to win in El Salvador, try as Moriah and I might. Evelyn, who doled my glorious push, wins the qualifying points for London. By the middle of the week, however, there is something unexpected I've won—a respect for trying among the peloton of my competitors, their nods and smiles a fleeting homage to the Empress of Maybe. Even without points, I've found small gains in the confidence that comes in recognizing one's self-improvement. It is perhaps one of the most thrilling moments in an athlete's life when we cross the quiet barrier of wondering about our potential into finally realizing it. Maybe that's where the points, literal and figurative, lie in wait.

A PIRATE'S LIFE FOR ME
April 2009

I'VE SPENT THE PAST FOUR NIGHTS sleeping with Johnny Depp. I'm exhausted. Alas, it isn't Depp who's worn me out but the 150 female cyclists I've been racing against over the past week. This doesn't explain Depp, but I'm getting there.

My teammates and I are racing the San Dimas Stage Race and Redlands Bicycle Classic, two of the most high-profile bike races in the States, set just outside Los Angeles. Stage races are extremely strenuous multi-day cycling competitions that sound like a good idea while signing up, but not so much during the event. They hurt. Bad. But it's a good bad. While cycling offers rewards such as extreme fitness and the thrill of victory, there are also crashes, road rash, and mind-numbing physical exertion that borders on delirium. Apparently, we elite riders find this fun. Or perhaps we have deep-seated emotional issues stemming back to childhood, or we are the product of genetic wiring that leaves us little choice in our definitions of "fun." No one really knows what drives a person into the world of cycling, but the ones that stick around truly love it uncon-ditionally. Especially the female racers.

While most men's pro teams have large budgets and corporate sponsors, the women are still working their way up the ladder of global recognition. For the majority of elite

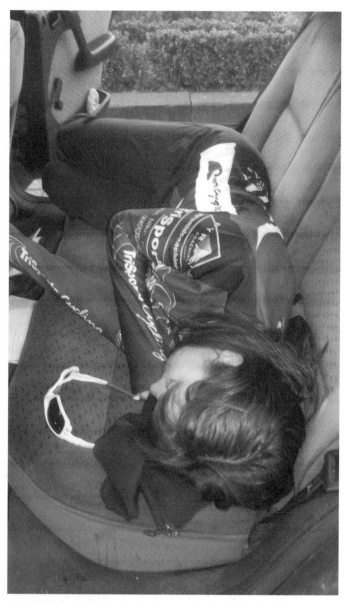

April 2009. Backseats of cars and beds of strangers; how female pro cyclists roll.

female racers, that means taking a no-frills approach to the sport. Flying to events is a luxury. Most of us drive to races, playing road trip games such as, "How many cyclists can you stuff in a Volkswagen?" Even in the elite ranks, we often pay for our meals and gas out of our pockets, and we're lucky (and grateful) when team managers/owners cover entry fees and the occasional dinner. Our bikes are usually corporate brand-name loaners, as the irony of the sport is that most elite cyclists can't afford their own stellar carbon-fiber machines at retail price. Then there's the lodging. Hotels during stage races are usually not in the women's race budget, so we rely on homestays to keep us sheltered. And Johnny Depp to keep us warm.

Homestays are local families near race venues who kindly agree to take in pro athletes for free. We use their kitchens to cook our prerace meals and sleep on their beds, couches, and floors. For this trip, my Trisports Cycling teammate, Marilyn, and I are assigned a homestay with a family in Redlands, California. Marilyn and I share the room of the family's 4-year-old son, who is in turn relocated to the living room couch. Thanks to SpongeBob's absorbing presence on the living room TV, this transition goes remarkably smoothly. His 2-year-old sister, however, recently borrowed my laptop for a game of "Let's sled down the stairs." Marilyn claims the futon in the 4-year-old's room. I take the kid's bed, which is a replica of a pirate ship—sails and all—complete with a *Pirates of the Caribbean* bedspread starring Depp's dingy and disheveled Jack Sparrow character.

After the first day of racing in the four-day event at the Redlands Bicycle Classic, I find myself a bit further back in the time trial results than I had hoped. This is bike racing:

sometimes you soar, sometimes you suck, sometimes you settle somewhere in between. And when you're physically exhausted, mentally dejected, and in a strange bed far from home, sometimes you question everything. I whisper to my nap-dozing teammate:

"Marilyn?"

"Hmmm."

"I'm 34 years old, and I'm asleep in a pirate ship bed of a 4-year-old, neither of which belongs to me. Is this weird?"

"Kind of."

"Aren't I supposed to have a 4-year-old?"

"Probably."

"How did I get here?"

Marilyn laughs. She knows I'm not referring to my decade-old Volvo wagon with 153,000 miles that got us (barely) to southern California from Tucson.

"We love bike racing?" she suggests.

"Right," I say. "Thanks." I turn over, considering this truth. I do love this racing life, as bizarre, exhausting, and underfunded as it is. I especially love how it found me, suddenly and wholly, gripping me for one reason and refusing to let go for another.

As a sports journalist and elite athlete, I was offered an assignment in 2006 by ESPN. The company wanted me to investigate what it takes to get to the Olympic Games. The catch? I was both the reporter and the guinea pig. For two years, I attempted to qualify for the Beijing Summer Olympics in road cycling. While I had a short career as a mediocre pro triathlete (and an MFA in creative writing in my back pocket), the assignment alone wasn't quite enough to get me to Beijing. Oddly, though, after two years of road cycling, I came quite close. Too close. When my project with ESPN concluded in 2008, my love of cycling did not. In fact, it grew—and so did my muscles, ability, and results. I decided to shoot for the 2012 Games, which is why three years after ESPN, I'm in a boat-shaped kiddie bed in a stranger's house setting sail with the Pirates of the Caribbean and a plastic flask of electrolytes dribbling near the headboard. Two more years of racing may just float me to the shores of England.

Or it might not. Like most women in their early thirties, I've done some thinking about my life path. I've compared the "What I've got" list with the "What I thought I'd have by now" list. Here's a brief rundown:

What I Thought I'd Have at 34:
Husband
Kids
Stable career
Dog
Cute wardrobe
A steady routine
Predictability
Happiness

What I actually have at 34:
Singledom
Bicycles
Freelance work
Cactus
Farmer's tan
Spontaneity
Stories
Happiness

Strange how the road to happiness can take such different routes. Occasionally we all suffer from GrassIsGreener-Itis, thinking we want or need the things our conventional peers have. Sometimes the cycling life makes me angry, annoyed, and inconvenienced. But for the most part, it brings me great joy. I often live out of a suitcase, but I also get to live in the moment. I have to be on my best behavior in homestay settings. But I meet wonderful, interesting people. I worry if I'll make ends meet. But I am getting by. I don't know where this cycling life will lead. But no one knows where any life will lead. I decide that's enough thinking for one night.

Sometimes—especially during a stage race—it is best to remember that not all life questions need to be terribly deep.

"Marilyn?" I whisper.

"Hmmm."

"Do you think Johnny Depp is hot?"

"Yeah. But not so much as a pirate."

"Aye," I agree. But I'm glad he's here with me, anyway.

Q AND A:
WHAT'S IT LIKE TO BE A CYCLIST?
July 2011

AS A COMPETITIVE CYCLIST, I get a lot of questions from curious non-cyclists who wonder what it takes—and why anyone would want—to do the things we do. Long hours in the saddle, prize money in the hundreds (not thousands or millions), little recognition, unflattering clothing, risks of crashing, ethics of cheating…the curiosity about cycling's intricacies is endless. The overall answer is simple; when you love your sport, you simply overlook the difficulties. But it is human nature for others to wonder about those difficulties and about what it takes to be an elite athlete. Below are the top 10 questions I've been asked most over the years of my cycling life and the answers, which, of course, are completely valid, accurate, and morally sound. Ish.

1: How many miles did you ride today?
A: One hundred miles. This is often a blatant lie. Instead, I average the daily miles I've ridden since someone last asked how many miles I've ridden, and that is usually about 100. Explaining to a non-cyclist about interval workouts, sprint training, climbing repeats, long rides vs. short rides, and how cyclists usually don't go by miles but by time, intensity,

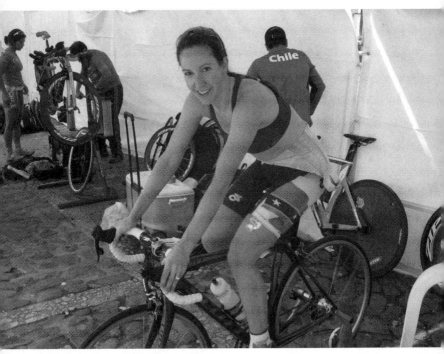

"How far did you ride today?" Not far enough to escape that question.

recovery, and other factors specific to the day and an upcoming event usually results in glazed eyes and an unspoken regret for asking. If I tell people I did an 8.9-kilometer mile prologue interval averaging more than 300 watts, they only hear "eight miles" and neglect to understand the distance may be short but the effort causes a feeling of bleeding from one's eyeballs and internal combustion of the spleen. But if I tell people I rode 100 miles, they say, "Oooh" and seem to appreciate/comprehend large round numbers.

2: Are you going to be in, or have you ever been in, the Olympics?

A: Alas, that's a question only fate, time, and Google can answer.

3: Do you have a very strict diet?

A: Yes. I am very strict with food. It is not uncommon to find me standing in front of an open fridge and disciplining the groceries in a Scottish Fat Bastard accent to "Get in my belly!" or to ask others if they're going to finish whatever is on their plate and if not, may I have it.

4: Do you think Lance cheated?

A: Evelyn Stevens. Marianne Vos. Emma Pooley. Lizzie Armistead. Kristin Armstrong.

Huh?

Those are just five of the hundreds of female pro cyclists who deserve more attention and discussion than the question of whether Lance cheated. Pick one. I'll tell you all about her.

5: Aren't you afraid of being hit by a car?

A: I'm far more afraid of a sedentary life.

6: Have you ever crashed?

A: (A nod to indicate "yes.") Cyclists don't like this question. Superstition, karma, and odds require us to change the subject quickly and offer only nonverbal affirmation that the gods of jinx cannot hear. We'd rather you'd ask us if we've ever won a race.

7: Have you ever won a race?

A: Yes, I totally dominated the Category 4s.

What's a Category 4?
It's, uh, the first step in becoming an Olympian.
Oh, good for you!
Thank you so much!

8: This is embarrassing, but I just have to know: What happens if you have to pee in the middle of a long race?

A: If it is a one-day race, you either hold it or you go in your shorts. If it is a multi-day stage race where the distances often require four-plus hours of riding and constant hydration is a must, sometimes there is a "natural break" mid-race. Usually, the race leader will ride easy for a few minutes while women pull over and pee on the side of the road. Obviously, this "break" is not during a critical time in the race, and any rider who chooses to attack is reprimanded and blackballed—anyone who survived high school knows it's not a good idea to piss off multiple groups of females. Those are the options: pull over and pee on the roadside, or don't pull over and pee in your shorts. In the case of the latter, it is polite to go to the back of the peloton first.

9: How old are you?
A: 38.

So how much longer do you plan to ride? I assume you want to have children soon?

A: Would you have asked me either of those questions if I were a dude?

10: Why do you do this sport? What is it about cycling you like so much?

A: For the long answer, search *As Good as Gold*. There

are many social, physical, and psychological answers in my book for why I do what I do as a 30-plus-year-old athlete. But for the shorter version, I'm going to let my 7-year-old self answer why I like racing bicycles, which still holds true today: *I like to get on my bike and see how fast I can make it go. The wind feels good on my face.*

THE ART OF GETTING BY
October 2012

FOR MOST FEMALE professional cyclists, their story starts something like this: Girl meets bike. Girl loves bike. Girl gets fast. Pro team likes girl. Pro team offers small salary. Girl must work and race simultaneously.

Boy, that's tough. Here's how girl does it.

Mary Zider of Team Colavita came to cycling the way most U.S. pro riders do—through a background of non-cycling-related sports.

"At a very young age I was always being dragged by older sisters to run the track or do some crazy workout in our yard," said Zider, who grew up in Barre, Vermont. She never resisted the dragging, and the sibling workout sessions instilled in her an early passion for soccer, basketball, and lacrosse. After a soccer career at Boston College and qualifying for the Boston Marathon, Zider—who'd grown used to a schedule of training and competition—craved an athletic outlet to fill the void.

"I started riding with some friends and joined a local cycling group called the Crack O Dawn, which trained at 5:45 AM, and quickly realized this was my next competitive adventure," Zider said. As she completed her senior year, majoring in human development focusing on human re-source management, she knew she wanted to cycle at a

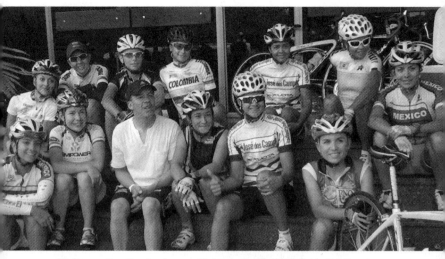

Working overtime. How female pros get it done as the UCI drags its feet on instating a base salary rule for women's pro cycling.

high level. She knew that to do that, she'd need a flexible schedule or a unique job. Zider took positions at Boston College's graduate school admissions office and at Beaver Country Day School in nearby Brookline, as well as manning the counter at a boutique fitness studio.

"I was able to work jobs that provided some flexibility, but the hours within my day became so structured that any error such as an unexpected appointment or a traffic hold-up could be detrimental to my training," said Zider, who acknowledged that pro cycling training often requires upward of 20 hours of workouts a week. "[Work] became very stressful, and training for a long-term race wasn't something I could sustain with the few hours of sleep I was getting. I was quickly burning out."

The dream of racing professionally was worth it, despite

the physical toll, and Zider had the will to find a way to make it all happen.

"My determination and work ethic kept me in sight of my goals," she said. "It has taken years to find that right job situation, but I can now proudly say I am very fortunate to have a job that supplements my racing profession and allows me to pursue my love and passion for cycling."

Zider, who signed on with Team Colavita in 2012, took a customer-service position with Eastern Mountain Sports that allows her to work remotely. This aids her demanding physical training by lessening the time she spends standing or sitting for work.

"I only work about six or seven hours per day with no commute. This allows me to train the hours I need during the week and get those few extra hours of sleep that really make a difference," she said. "There is still a lot of juggling of schedules to make this whole racing thing work out, but for me it's been worth every minute."

While creating a chance to race professionally is an incredible achievement, especially now when a tough economy has made it difficult to secure sponsors, there are still hurdles. In women's cycling, the U.S. has fewer than seven fully funded pro teams. Only a select handful of cyclists earn a decent living from a combination of salaries, prize winnings, and endorsements. The majority of U.S. female racers earn well below the poverty-line income of $11,170 for a single-person household. Couple that with any unforeseen setbacks, and the dream of racing professionally becomes extremely fragile.

For Zider, whose income from EMS and cycling was intended to supplement her household, a crisis arose when her boyfriend became unemployed.

"At that time, his salary was pretty much our primary source of income," she said. "This period of life was very challenging and stressful. It would have been very comforting to know that, as a pro racer, I would have a regular salary that was comparable to other female pro sports or to men's cycling base salaries, but unfortunately that is many years away."

Like Zider, other pro cyclists have found a way to merge their careers with their athletic passions, but working two careers is far from ideal for any athlete. Former U.S. time trial champion Alison Powers, who races for NOW/Novartis for MS, uses her experience to guide other cyclists at her training company, ALP Cycles Coaching. While Powers can work from home, the time and focus on others required still hinders her training and racing schedule.

"As much as I enjoy coaching, it would be nice to not have to do it. It can get a little overwhelming dealing with bikes and training all day long, day after day," Powers admitted. "Even when I am at races, I have to take care of my athletes while they race. Sometimes, I'd rather sit on the couch, turn off my brain, and watch TV and let my body recover. But that doesn't happen. It doesn't happen for many women in sport."

Nicky Wangsgard, a 13-year veteran of pro cycling now racing for Primal/MapMyRide, is also a professor of special education at Southern Utah University where she works 30 to 40 hours a week. While SUU is supportive of Wangsgard's racing, her previous employers at another university were less than enthused. The pride of being an elite athlete was traded for secrecy and fear of losing her job.

"At the college I taught at before Southern Utah University, I was told that my colleagues would think I'm not a scholarly educator if I'm a bike racer," Wangsgard said. "So I kept my racing a secret. I'm lucky SUU is so supportive. My colleagues love reading my race reports and seeing photos of the finish or race action. If I need a class covered, there is always someone willing to help." Even with the support of her department, a 30-40-hour week is a difficult physical demand on Wangsgard.

"I've noticed that I do not get as much down time to recover [from workouts and races] as I would like. At times, I have to work out early in the morning right before work, which means I'm on my feet all day right after a hard workout. Or I'm on my feet all day and then working out tired and not feeling as strong as I could have felt," Wangsgard said.

Most female road cycling pros race from February to October, with the majority averaging 30 to 50 race days per year. For those competing internationally, the number of races can double. For Zider, months away from home were the norm.

"I found myself traveling on the road with very limited time at home between events, sometimes just long enough to do laundry," she said. "Once, we left for a mini training camp in the end of April, then it was off to the races, literally, until the end of July."

Yet despite the global growth in both strength and numbers for women's pro cycling, there is still no minimum salary for racers. In men's cycling, the neophyte pros on the UCI continental teams are guaranteed a base pay of $29,000. (For top men's professionals on the higher-ranking UCI WorldTour teams, the average salary jumps to $331,500.)

"If the top American female cyclists, let's say just 50 women, were paid half of the salary that the top 50 American men are paid, the women could possibly work part-time or not at all," Wangsgard said. "Most of my teammates who decided not to work have a hard time paying their bills. They are dependent on race winnings, which leaves them stressed and worried. Most of the female cyclists I know race because they love the sport, not because they are making a good living."

The love of sport, however, should not take a back seat to equality. Zider and Powers agree.

"It would be nice to see a minimum-salary agreement for all UCI women's teams," Zider said. "This would guarantee a rider a minimum salary in which [women cyclists] could plan and build a life around." Powers notes that small steps like having male cyclists recognize and champion the rights and accomplishments of female racers go a long way in bridging the equality gap. Until the day comes when cycling salaries are equal, most female racers find that a positive outlook helps keep everything in perspective.

"I decided long ago that happiness is more important than money," Powers said. "Therefore, I have only worked jobs that have provided me freedom to ride my bike."

For Zider, and for most women on the pro circuit, the decision to race despite the obstacles of income eventually comes down to love. "There are times when I stop and ask myself, 'Is it worth it?' But when I look at the memories, the friendships, and the experiences I've been able to have because of cycling, it becomes crystal clear why we do what we do. I love the feeling of pushing my body to its limit, always striving to be better and stronger. I ride and race my bike to enjoy the adventure."

As female riders continue to voice their opinions, rise through the ranks, and strive for equality, change is inevitable. Luckily, the heart of the story will ultimately stay the same: Girl meets bike. Girl loves bike. The end.

OF PIGEONS AND PRIZE MONEY
March 2011

STOP ME IF YOU'VE HEARD this one before.

A woman rides her bike past a house. A man in the front yard is speaking sternly to a pigeon. The woman stops and asks what the man is doing.

The man says, "I'm teaching the pigeon to race."

The woman asks, "Why?"

The man says, "Because pigeon racing earns 10 times the prize money as women's cycling! Ha, ha, ha!"

As a joke, this fails miserably. As reality, this scenario is miserably true. In Belgium, where I've been living and racing (bikes, not birds) for the past six weeks, I've been staying down the street from a man who races pigeons for a living. Pigeon racing is all the rage in Belgium and other parts of Europe where the birds are trained to fly long distances as quickly as possible. They're brought to a meeting place, released, and then the owners drive hundreds of miles to pick them up in Paris or Frankfurt or Brussels. Like in horse racing, wagers are placed and prize purses are lucrative for the fastest bird. The top pigeon can take home up to 10,000 Euros. That's about $16,000 for a bird to do what birds do best—fly from one place to another.

For a woman to ride her bicycle from Point A to Point B and get there before the rest of her flock, the prize money is rarely more than $1,000. And that's at a top-level UCI race. Yet that's not the worst part of the meager winnings. Because cycling is a team sport and most women's teams enter six to eight riders per event, that prize money is then divided by the number of people on the team. It's rare that the best women's racers in the world will take home more than a couple of hundred dollars per event—not even enough to buy a world-class pigeon.

Male cyclists, on the other hand, earn slightly more than the birds. At Paris-Roubaix, one of the most famous single-day events in cycling, the winner nets about $40,000 and the prize purse for the top 20 finishers pays out more than $120,000. Multi-day events known as stage races bring more capital gains, and the pinnacle event—the Tour de France—awards the winner nearly 800,000 Euros to split with his team. Of course, even this pales in comparison with the earnings of the top athletes in the world's other professional sports—baseball, football, golf, hockey, and basketball. Even cricket. Not the bug-racing kind of cricket, though I'm guessing if there is such a thing, those earnings probably top women's cycling, too.

The reality, of course, is that barely anyone in women's cycling does it for the money. We do it for the love of the sport, the thrill of racing, and the pride of living life to the fullest. In that manner, we're fabulously rich. But that doesn't mean we should settle for the inequalities. Equal prize money isn't the first step in our battle. Exposure and inclusion are the initial hurdles, as is media coverage. Eurosport runs nearly six hours of television coverage of the men's Tour of Flanders. At the end of the broadcast, a 20-second clip of the women's sprint to the finish line flashed by on the screen. The women don't even get invited to all the major events.

There is no Paris-Roubaix, there is no Tour de France, there is no internal push by the sport's governing body to have these races achieve parity for women. Meanwhile in the highly progressive aviary world, the boy pigeons and the girl pigeons are allowed to race the same event.

Change must come from within cycling's organization to give the athletes the equality they deserve. Somewhere along the way, the good ol' boys network of cycling has overlooked the fact that including women's coverage isn't just good for the athletes—it would likely double cycling's audience and any given event's sponsorship potential. Like the old Chinese proverb says, "Women hold up half the sky." We deserve our half of the road, as well.

I guarantee that if Christian Prudhomme, the director of the Tour de France, opened his event to pro women's teams and offered equal camera time and prize money, there would be 200 of the best female bike racers on the start line who would give the organization, sponsors, and cycling fans exactly what they want—an incredible bike race among the world's top athletes, regardless of gender. That's when our equality starts.

First, however, I should get back to my Olympic quest, where all the prize money in the world and all the pigeons on the planet can't buy me what I need most: Olympic qualification points. For now, that's the journey. I'll conquer the Tour de France next year. Prudhomme will need that time to prepare for me, anyway.

WANT TO RACE WITH LONG HAIR? FINE.
July 2009

"SAYS HERE YOUR NUMBER was folded," the head referee tells me.

"I don't fold my numbers," I say, turning to show her the back of my cycling jersey and the two gigantic yet neatly pinned race numbers, splayed across the expanse of my upper back in their entire, unfolded glory. I am number 282. Clearly says so, in what appears to be Times New Roman, 400-point font. Bold. Twice on my back and once on my bicycle.

"Hmmm," she says.

I am at the sign-in table of the Fitchburg Longsjo Classic bicycle race in Massachusetts, a four-day stage race celebrating its 50th anniversary. It's a wonderful event with marvelous competition and terrific organization—and slightly nearsighted refs. Today is Day 3, and on the sign-in sheet (where we are required to give our signature each day) my name is highlighted in fluorescent pink marker. So too are the names of four other female cyclists in the professional women's category. I roll my eyes, as things like fluorescent marker stripes, asterisks, or underlines are usually indicative of penalties, disqualifications, or fines. There is no penalty explanation written next to my day-glo name, and I am advised to check the wall. The referee points to a wall with sheets of paper taped to it. The wall

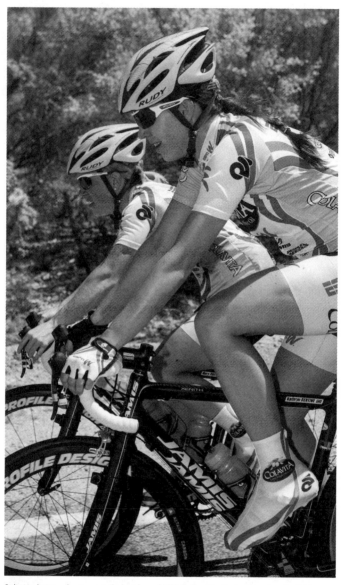

Splitting hairs—how ponytails, braids, and USA Cycling don't mix. (Jonathan Devich/
epicimages.us)

tells me that I am "in violation of rule 4H7a," but neither the wall nor the paper say any more.

"What is 4H7a?" I ask the ref. Random numbers and letters are another bad sign, and I immediately fear 4H7a is the H1N1 of the cycling rulebook.

"I don't know," she admits.

"Well, how much is the fine?"

"Twenty dollars."

I wrack my brain over yesterday's race details. Didn't cross the yellow lines. Didn't cause a crash. Didn't litter. Didn't cut the course. Didn't take EPO. Didn't use unsportsmanlike conduct. Didn't yell at a referee. (Yet). Didn't finish high enough in the results for anyone to really pay any attention to me at all. What the heck did I do? I turn and walk away, shaking my head. Hell, if I'm gonna pay a $20 fine when the ref doesn't even…

"Know what it is!" she calls after me. "Your hair. It's too long. Probably covered the number. That's an obstruction."

∘ ∘ ∘

In the bathroom near the race start, I take a handheld mirror and check out the back of my head. I have a low ponytail roped into a thin, tight braid. The ponytail is where it has to be, at the bottom of my scalp, as the mandatory helmet takes up the rest of my head's real estate. The very bottom of my braid barely even tickles the top border of one race number. I hunch up my shoulders, and lo! The braid lowers itself onto *half* of the first numeral, the first two, in 282. Seriously? Am I really being charged $20 for this…*obstruction*? I put my braid in a bun and race with the hairy knot in an uncomfortable, hot, snagging purgatory between my neck and helmet.

I am not a high-maintenance woman. I am a bike racer. Half of my life is spent in cycling clothing, which is often made for men. There are bugs in my hair, dirt on my face, lugies on my shoulder, and an unidentifiable layer of grime on my entire body for the majority of each day. I am okay with this. Just let me have my ponytail. Not because it's part of my personal identity of femininity, but because it isn't right to fine an athlete when the system is at fault.

o o o

Before we start taxing athletes for having long hair, we need to make sure that the error doesn't lie within the "obscured" system. Let's look at the paper race numbers. In the world of cycling, only U.S.-based events use race numbers that are double or triple the size of race numbers in other countries. All the other nations use small square numbers, usually 4" x 4". The two numbers are pinned on the back pockets of the jersey, which sit at the rider's waist/lower back where hair length is not an issue for men or women. Only in the U.S. do we have two enormous numbers, some measuring 5" x 8", which race directors require we attach to our upper backs. For any cyclist, let alone females, there's not a lot of upper back to begin with. Wear the numbers any lower, and they overlap—that's another fine. Sure, the huge, high-placed numbers are easier for refs to read. But with video playback at finish lines and multiple ways to tell professional cyclists apart (team jerseys, bike numbers, our faces, etc), and race numbers attached to our bike frames, I'm not sure we need two enormous sheets of paper pinned to our upper bodies.

So, why such a big size and placement discrepancy with our numbers? Because our supersized U.S.-manufactured race numbers include sponsor names and slogans. Instead of just "282," our race numbers also read "Fitchburg Longsjo Classic, 50th Anniversary" or "Citibank" or "Pete's Pasta Palace." That's a lotta room, a lotta paper. I'm all for sponsorship and advertising—our sport relies on it—but when it comes down to a rider getting a fine for not being a proper billboard, then something's wrong. My job is to race a bicycle. The refs' job is to make sure we do it fairly. Not to hand out fines for ponytails. A race director might argue that my particular fine had nothing to do with the sponsor logos being covered by my ponytail but that my actual number was obstructed at the moment I crossed the finish line. Okay. Well, in the event that half-a-digit of my three-digit, 400-point font number plastered onto three different parts of my bicycle and me that was viewable to three different refs and also reviewable on video camera, might not be legible...there's still a commonsense factor missing. All of the women in the race were given numbers in the 200s. Just as all the pro men had numbers in the 100s or lower. So, even though the last two (highly visible) digits of my number "-82" should have sufficed just fine to deduce I was female rider 282, there were three other context clues that clearly could have helped out those refs who were confused by my "obscured" number:

a) I'm in a race surrounded by women.

b) I am a woman.

c) *I have a ponytail.*

As for rule 4H7a, the USA Cycling rulebook decrees any "number or frameplate altered, mutilated, badly positioned, or covered at the finish" is entitled to a first-offense fine of $20. Next offense, $35, and third strike and you're out via disqualification. Technically, if my number only covered one-sixth of my total race number, I should only pay $3.33.

But I went ahead and sent USA Cycling a check for the whole $20. Otherwise I'm not allowed to race. Please USA Cycling, please leave my ponytail alone. I love the races you sponsor, the events you hold, the guidance you give, the athletes you support, and the way with which you conduct 99 percent of your business. You look out for your members in so many regards. If the braids and the numbers don't mix, the numbers should be trimmed before the hair—or simply worn lower on the body like the rest of the world. It isn't a crime to have long hair. Also, a large number of the women's pro field—regardless of hair length—struggle physically and financially just to attend your races. Twenty-dollar fees may not be so much to your organization, but for some of us athletes, that is an entire stage race food budget. Keep fining the riders who cross the yellow lines, who break the rules, and who act less than sportsmanlike. But come on. Don't fine us for our hair. That's the true obstruction.

A CYCLIST'S LETTER TO SANTA
December 2011

DEAR SANTA,

Despite the fact I am roughly 30 years too old to be writing you, thought I'd get in touch. Santa, I'm pretty lucky not to be in need of anything tangible. I've got health, happiness, and love, so I'm all set in the universal sense. Unless you happen to be buddies with the head of the IOC and the UCI (Union Cycliste Internationale) and can put in a good word for me during my Olympic qualification attempt this year in road cycling. Still, I'm pretty sure that's a whole different kind of gift and one I'm likely responsible for on my own.

Instead of presents under the tree, I thought I'd ask you for some mental and emotional gifts this year. See, 2012 is coming up and it is gonna be a toughie—in the worthwhile sense—as I shoot for a spot at the Games. I'm not sure if you have any magic sprinkle dust that takes care of minor mental woes, but if you do, my Christmas wish is that you pepper some of it into my oatmeal or make it into some new-fangled fancy peanut butter. Any medium is acceptable, though a syringe might raise eyebrows. Here's my wish list:

1. Watts. I could use more watts. The ones I have are pretty good, but if you have some extras lying around the workshop, I'll most happily take them.

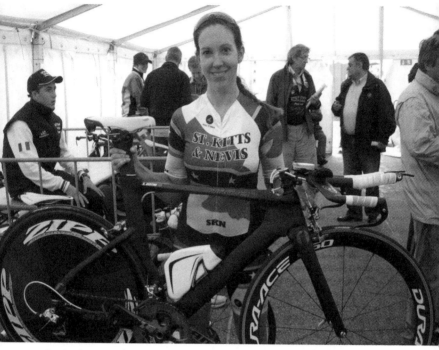

I've already got a bike, Santa. Can you please bring me a wooden club and special pants?

2. New pants. One of my former competitors, 2008 U.S. criterium and road race national champion Brooke Miller, once gave me some really good advice about bike racing. She said that before I get to the start line of a race, I need to put on my "F--- You" Pants. Apparently these help an athlete focus on her goals and do a lot to intimidate the competition. I think these pants are metaphorical, but if you have any in stock, I'll take a medium. Seven pairs of them.

3. The UCI has a rule that the majority of the riders on a professional women's team must have a racing age

of less than 28 years old. In a sport like cycling, where many women peak (and win world and Olympic titles) in their mid-thirties—well, this backdated rule isn't helping women sustain careers in the sport. Wondering if you could sprinkle a dose of reality to the UCI.

4. TV time for female athletes. Santa, this one is not specific to cycling, but to all women athletes and teams in the majority of sports. For the love of Rudolph, can you please rewire the minds of our TV execs with an "If you build it, they will come" mentality? If they take a leap of faith and broadcast women's sports in a manner that educates and excites, they will be rewarded with a larger audience and higher ratings. If they don't know how do to this, please have them call me. I have a black belt in Getting Things Done.

5. Stupidity. Likely something not often requested as a gift, I'm looking for a little extra stupidity this year. Not that I don't have plenty of my own; the problem is, I tend to think too much in races. I wonder what others are doing, worry about the ifs and whens of attacks and counterattacks, and question whether or not I can do this or that. I'd really like to see what my body can do without my head getting in the way. Do you have something that could turn my brain off for a few hours a day? Perhaps a pocket-size wooden club?

6. Have your elves invented a bicycle that doesn't revert a cyclist's posture to that of a Paleolithic knuckle-dragger? I used to get compliments on my posture. After five years on the bike, I'm about one genome away from Igor.

7. If possible, could you sprinkle some magic dust on athletes who take performance-enhancing drugs so that they spontaneously combust mid-race? That would be cool, Santa.

8. I'm trying really hard to enjoy yoga. I suppose I am asking you to bring me patience, or reduce my competitive urge to knock over the 80-year-old who can touch his toes. What a show-off.

9. In my attempt to race for Olympic points, it is nearly impossible to get to all of the qualifiers. If you're not using your sled for 364 days of the year, could I borrow it to reach some of my races? Or, if you're more comfortable doing the driving, I'll reimburse you for the…reindeer hay. Either way, it would be cheaper than flying Delta. Thanks, Santa.

10. Finally Big Red, I'd like to ask you for one last thing. I should probably ask you for superhuman strength or the ability to win races or multiple trips to the UCI podiums next year. You'd probably tell me all that potential stuff is already inside me. In that case, I'd like to ask you for a map. I know my potential is in there, too, and I will try to find it with the pocket-sized club, but if you have a map of my head, heart, and future, that would be most handy. If not, that's okay. I'll figure it out with my newfound stupidity. But man, I could really use the pants, watts, and sled.

Thanks for reading, and Merry Christmas, Santa. Hope you, the wife, and abundant family of tiny people and odd pets are doing great.

Your fan,

Kathryn

BELGIUM BOUND
February 2011

BELGIUM IS IMPOSSIBLE not to love; a diverse country that gave the world chocolate, waffles, Jean Claude Van Damme, and the Smurfs. And of course, a passion for cycling, which is why I'm here.

For pro and elite cyclists, racing in Belgium is much like getting a tetanus shot—painful but ultimately for our benefit. Races here boast huge participant fields, tiny streets, pavement from the Middle Ages, and scary corners that demand the competition to be fearless and hyper-vigilant. I've come to Belgium for two reasons: to make myself a better cyclist and hopefully win some Olympic qualification points. The latter is rather difficult, as often 200 women show up to the start line, and qualification points go only to the top eight finishers. My optimistic side argues that someone has to be in the top eight, so there's still a chance. My realistic side laughs openly at my optimism.

I arrive in Belgium in early March. In most cases, top-level cyclists don't worry too much about the logistics of racing. The travel is covered, hotels or homestays are provided, and their biggest focus is to show up and race. My path's a little different. Because the St. Kitts and Nevis cycling federation isn't backed by a nationally funded budget, getting to my races is mostly funded out of pocket. But

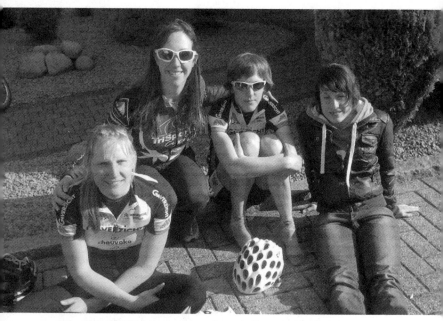

With my Dutch and Belgian teammates on Gaverzicht Matexi. No really, they're psyched to have me. Promise.

getting into races is even harder, a skill that calls for three main ingredients: honesty, luck, and Google Translate.

With the majority of the Spring UCI (Union Cycliste Internationale) races held in Belgium and neighboring Holland, my first step was to email every race director in these two countries if I could race their events in March and April. I told them my story, that I'm the national time trial and road race champion of St. Kitts and Nevis, looking to gain qualification points for the 2012 Olympics. Actually, I don't tell them anything, my translator does. Sometimes the translator is a friend or a stranger I find on Twitter or Facebook, sometimes it is via Google Translate. I send out hundreds of emails and hope a few race directors respond. If I'm lucky enough to get a response, it is usually this: "You must be on a local team to race our events." My next email asks if they can help me find a local team. And so the back-and-forth emails ensue, in foreign languages, with my Olympic dreams hanging in the delicate balance of strangers.

Another reason to love Belgium—it has wonderful strangers. A positive response from a Belgian race director gets me in touch with a local team, and before I know it, I'm into seven races as part of Team Gaverzicht Matexi of Deerlijk, Belgium. Better still, the race director finds me a place to stay within his extended family.

My host family, Els and Wilfried, live just a mile from the start line of my first race. They have taken me in for six weeks, providing me with food and shelter and, most importantly, conversation and companionship. It is one thing to go forth into the world and give it your all. It's another thing to do so when you're far from home and the comforting familiarity of my three main training staples: English, local roads, and peanut butter.

o o o

Three days off the plane, I enter my first race in Belgium, the Oomloop van het Hageland, which roughly translates into Tour of Unfamiliar People, Places, and Four Crashes in the First Hour. I don't speak Dutch, but I do speak cycling, so the translation proves mostly accurate. I also do not speak kilometer, but I am quickly learning. As it turns out, constantly asking my Belgian competitors, "How much farther, Papa Smurf?" isn't as much fun for them as it is for me.

Also not fun—chafing. A cardinal rule of cycling is never wear new bike shorts in a race without first washing them and breaking them in. New seams and different stitching patterns can wreak havoc Down Below. Luckily, there is a product for this discomfort. DZ Nuts is a glorious salve one uses to ease the wrath of fabric—bike seat—muscle friction. But, I have forgotten mine, and my Belgian team hands me a brand new pair of shorts just before the start. Halfway into the four-hour race, I can feel the new seams sawing their merciless welts into my nether region. Jean Claude Van *Damn* that hurts.

As it turns out, I don't make the top eight in my first race or the next eight or the next. Instead, I learn about the vicious three-minute rule. On the last lap of our 75-mile race—when I am just six miles from the finish and feeling pretty happy about avoiding the four crashes, surviving the cobblestone miles, and doing it all with razor seams lumberjacking my womanhood—strong Belgian winds and 39-degree temperatures take a toll on the peloton. Gaps begin to form, the cyclists start to crumble, and as I fight to keep contact with the peloton, I lose my battle against the wind. This is called blowing up—when all energy is sapped and a racer has nothing left. *Okay,* I decide. *That's OK for today. First race. Still a little jet lagged. Just roll it in and finish. Half the field's blown anyway. You're not alone.* That is when I learn Belgium doesn't really have a soft spot for finishing. Once a rider falls back from the peloton by three minutes, they're pulled from the course. This is like going to the New York City Marathon and setting up a thanks-for-coming-but-you-can-go-home-now detour for anyone slower than three hours. Today I am one of 90 (out of 196) competitors chopped from the finish with just six miles to go.

Still, at the finish, locals are saying "Congratulations!" to me. "For what?" I ask, bewildered they are congratulating a cut rider. "For making it as far as you did!" they say. I then learn I was the last rider cut, and had I been about 30 seconds faster, I would have been able to finish. I make a mental note to ask DZ Nuts if they have any product that eases brain friction. At the same time, I understand this sport well enough by now to know that no matter how strong, how prepared, and how willing an athlete is, sometimes we all blow up. The upside? It's impossible to blow up and *not* come back stronger the next week. Well, maybe the week after that. Regardless, I have 14 months to go, and you can bet your waffles I'm getting better, faster, and stronger in Belgium.

∘ ∘ ∘

I am working on my inner bitch. My mental trash talk. My me-first-get-out-of-my-way-ness. Because if I don't get in touch with Aggressive Kathryn, I won't survive racing in Belgium. Racing here is different than in the U.S. For starters, European races have three or four times as many racers as the majority of our U.S. events. It isn't so much the 200 riders gathered at the start line that freaks me out; it's the fact that, in Belgium, there seems to be a racing discrepancy on a molecular level. When the gun goes off (which, by the way, is preceded by no fanfare or warning), these women don't simply try to move around one another, they vie to occupy the same exact molecules of space as myself and my bike.

Despite the fact we might have a four-hour race, the peloton sprints to more than 27 mph at the start. Riders look to position themselves at the front because everyone knows what's coming: itty-bitty European roads the size of American sidewalks. Getting too far back is dangerous. If a crash happens—excuse me, *when* a crash happens—anyone stuck behind it is bottlenecked out of contention for the win. Hence, the fight to infiltrate the personal atomic space of others proves necessary. And frightening.

It's not that I'm a pushover. I have plenty of inner bitch. Just ask my husband about my lovely habit of screaming at the TV every time an actor uses bad grammar. The problem is channeling this emotion when I'm on the bike. Actually, not on the bike, but in the peloton. I do just fine without 200 people around me. As a time trial specialist, my strength comes in beating myself into mental and physical oblivion for an hour of solo riding where my opponent is a clock. A clock situated nicely on the sideline that respects my atomic existence. But that does me little good in my Olympic quest. There is no Olympic time trial qualification system for small countries such as St. Kitts and Nevis, which is new to cycling and doesn't have a previous Olympic berth. Any "new" country trying to get a cyclist to the Games must qualify that athlete via road-racing criteria, even if the athlete is a time trial racer. So I find myself among 200 giant foreign ladies, all of whom appear to know the formula for splitting atoms, as the one woman who only knows that *atom* is a noun.

My efforts of aggression are sincere. I get to the start line early. I seek out good wheels to follow. I put my elbows out and keep my insecurities in. But then it happens. A rider coming up on my right begins to invade my space. I force my handlebars ahead of hers. She forces hers ahead of mine. As our atoms collide via shoulder bumping, we can read each other's minds. *I want my win*, she thinks. "I want my mommy," I cry. And in that split second of doubt, when I think about how much I love the skin on my legs, I let the rider into the space ahead of me. This would not be such a problem if she didn't bring 30 of her closest friends with her.

For the next 20 minutes, I take lessons in what I call the Accordion School for Cyclists. I shoot to the back of the peloton, then try to compress myself up to the front, then get squeezed to the back, then to the front, and back again, all of which uses an exorbitant amount of energy and feels about as good as an accordion sounds. Finally, my inner bitch gets some nerve and whispers, "Hey, grammar police, you having a good time back here? Because if you're not, we could go home and watch *Glee* reruns and give up these silly Olympic dreams." That's when I remember there is only one thing greater than the knowledge of splitting atoms: reverse psychology.

In my third race since arriving in Europe, I finally finished ahead of the time cut, situated in the chase group not far behind the main pack. But I still need to be much farther up in the peloton to win Olympic points. I've learned, though, that before anyone moves up in any area of life, we first need to find our aggression, atoms, luck, the will to improve, and a hearty dose of inner glee. Okay Belgium, teach me all your cycing secrets.

THE SNELHEIDSMETER
February 2011

IN A GROUND-BREAKING training session in the small Belgian village of Tielt-Winge, I discovered evidence that will reverse the findings of decades of psychological research. Frowning, it turns out, can make you faster, stronger, and happier. And I have proof.

In the late winter of 2011, I lived and raced in Belgium for five weeks, away from my home, husband, friends, and teammates, in order to gain European race experience and help prepare for Olympic qualification events. In an unfamiliar country where I did not speak the language, I trained alone for hours, captivated by the scenery and solitude. I spent a fair amount of time getting lost. I met interesting people. I tried new foods. I saw castles and moats. I tried hard to look up at the world whizzing by me, a lost art among the modern-day training codes beckoning cyclists to stare down at one's stem-mounted Garmin, forever glued to our watts and power output. I, too, am guilty of staring at small screens, but in Belgium I tried to find creative ways to keep the big picture in check.

On a cold, gray, rain-spitting day (which was the February norm), I had a sprint interval session scheduled for the middle of my three-hour ride: two sets of five sprints, each sprint lasting 15-20 seconds. A 15-second sprint does

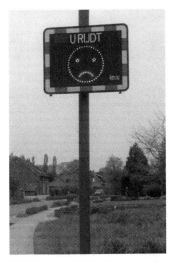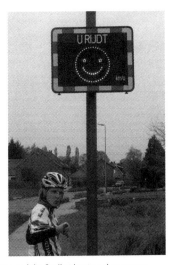

Tielt-Winge, Belgium. My buddy, Alison Testroete, and the Snelheidsmeter, the greatest training tool never invented.

not sound like much, but after hours of racing, that final intensity in the homestretch of a race is often all that matters for the win. Not a sprinter by nature, such workouts call for deeper motivation. Sprinting is also a bear of a workout to do alone, as outsprinting your shadow is far less appealing than racing someone else's. I was sulking a little heading into this particular workout. I had been feeling a little homesick, a little run down, a little frownypants, and I really had no desire or energy to do a sprint session that day. That's when I saw the *snelheidsmeter*.

The *snelheidsmeter* is a speed-sensing sign that flashes how many kilometers per hour a car is traveling. A few of the flat, fast, speed-enticing stretches of the residential streets in Tielt-Winge had *snelheidsmeters* installed, but I hadn't paid them much mind until today. The best part of the contraption is that between the flashing kilometer digits, a digital smiley face donning a bright green smile appears if the driver is at the correct speed. If a car triggers 50 kph (31 mph), the face frowns and the mouth turns red, visually disapproving of the driver. Over 75 kph, the smiley face gives the finger. Okay, that is not true. But it should be. I giggled as I went past the *snelheidsmeter* then realized the sign's speed sensor picks up bikes, too. I swung a quick U-turn. I had found the greatest sprint workout ever.

For the next 20 minutes, I did my best to turn that smile upside down. Old *snelly* and I battled it out for frown control. While the road was flat, the robust Belgian headwind kept the challenge lively—39 kph, 42 kph, then, on my final sprint…63 kph! Snelly finally frowns, I finally smile! Wow, 63 kph? I'd really improved. Only I hadn't…a Fiat sped by, and likely triggered the frown while I sprinted. I frown, snelly smiles. Do over. I lost track of the intervals, going above and beyond the necessary number my coach prescribed. I made it all the way up to 48 kph on my last attempt in the wind but couldn't quite convert the mood of the happy speed meter. My mood, however, altered tremendously—a great reminder of the power of perspective and the joy of breaking routines and how to go about finding a little inspiration in unexpected places. Sometimes trying to frown is a step in the right direction.

March in Belgium brought the arrival of the Canadian national team, and some (live!) people for me to train with. I brought my new Canadian friend, Alison Testroete, to race the *snelheidsmeter*. Alison, a veteran racer, didn't find the moody speed sensor nearly as amusing as I did, but we both agreed the opportunity to live, race, and experience foreign cultures while chasing an athletic dream is indeed something to smile about. As we headed back through town, I looked out over the blooming pear orchards of springtime in Belgium. Flowers are opening. Moats are flowing. Cyclists are everywhere. Street signs are smiling. If only Snelly could measure a life well lived, I would have short circuited that sucker from a mile away.

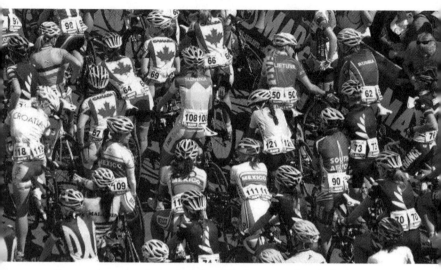

The women's pro peloton is comprised of incredibly diverse personalities. And bodies.
(Chris Tsorotes)

IN IT WITH ALL HER HEART
April 2012

IN MY ATHLETIC CAREERS ranging from figure skating to rowing to triathlon to cycling, I've trained and competed with men, women, gays, lesbians, blind, deaf, young, old, children, and athletes with less limbs and more guts than most people have. So when a cycling teammate of mine at the UCI Energiewacht Tour in Holland pointed out Natalie Van Gogh across the dining hall, saying, "That's Natalie. She used to be a he." My initial thought was, *Huh. That's a new one.*

New, at least, in my personal competitive experience. Transgendered athletes are rare but not exactly new in sport. The LPGA's Lana Lawless, tennis player Renee Richards, and most recently Washington University's women's hoops player Kai Allums—all transsexual athletes—have struggled for equality and caused many a question mark for the governing bodies of their sports. Other athletes, like South African track star Caster Semenya, (not transgendered but hermaphrodite), carry both the male and female chromosomes and are constantly questioned about their testosterone levels.

At first, I wasn't sure how I felt about the presence of a transgendered athlete in women's cycling. I had some questions about power, strength, and physical advantages. In the dining hall where dozens of women's cycling teams gathered for dinner during the four-day UCI Energiewacht Tour, Van Gogh's team was seated at a table next to mine. At 6'1", with a lean cyclist's body, a long chiseled face, a pony-tail of tight auburn curls, and solid muscular limbs, Van Gogh's physicality stands out among the other cyclists. She has the build and facial structure more typical of males. In terms of demeanor, she blended in with the rest of us. Eating dinner at her team's table, she talked quietly with her teammates, smiled often, and carried herself like any other dignified athlete: proud but without ostentation. She did not draw attention to herself, though curious eyes and quiet whispers followed Van Gogh from other tables.

"She's had the full operations," my teammate informed me, "so she races with the women now."

In cycling, where there is a definite physical difference between the high-end sprint power output of top male and female racers, I couldn't help but wonder if Natalie

Van Gogh was dominating the female field of competitors. Surely, despite the surgeries, she still has certain levels of testosterone that natural-born females don't possess? And her muscles, they still resemble those of a man, so they must add a power-to-weight ratio the rest of us females might not have? I mean, is she winning by landslides? I asked my teammates, also Dutch riders, what they thought of Van Gogh's presence in women's racing. The feelings were mixed. No one had a problem with Natalie as a person, but the issue of hormones came up. Transgendered athletes are supposed to ingest the hormones of their "new" sex. But what happens if a man who has transgendered to a woman stops taking her estrogen hormones? Then the athlete has more testosterone, which could be seen as an advantage. But this, like any kind of hormone therapy or drug use, is a private matter known only by the individual. No athlete will ever truly know if one of their competitors is taking hormones or not, unless they witness it.

Fascinating. Here we are in a sport constantly plagued by doping and steroid scandals usually involving male athletes taking testosterone supplements, and in the case of Natalie Van Gogh, her competitors hope she is taking her estrogen hormones. As it turns out, the International Olympic Committee is curious about such matters, too. Recently, the IOC ruled transgendered athletes and other women who test in the male range for functional testosterone must have their levels regulated if their testosterone percentages come in too high. There are all sorts of moral implications involved with the testing. Some feel it's sexist. Others think it's an intrusion of privacy. Many think the testing is a good idea. It is, without question, debatable territory.

As I see it, testing should be done in all cases where there is a potential for cheating, regardless of gender. If elite athletes need to be tested for any drugs that alter hormone levels or red blood cell count—whether natural or ingested—this has to apply for transgendered athletes as well as non-transgendered athletes.

I asked my teammate how Van Gogh was doing in the Dutch races and if she is dominating the podium in a manner in which other female competitors cannot keep up.

"Well, she's not quite winning the major events. But she's close. She does place highly, maybe top 15 or 20 in our races," my teammate said. While only the top three riders make the podium in cycling, prize money often goes 20 places deep in European races, and field sizes can grow to more than 200 competitors. In addition to prize money, those in the top 20 also catch the eye of professional team managers—a much-coveted source of attention in women's cycling where pro team contracts are extremely difficult to land. Also up for grabs in the top 8-to-12 places in stage races is another rare treasure: Olympic qualification points via UCI rankings. (Union Cyclist Internationale is the governing body of elite women's cycling). The more points a rider gets in UCI rankings, the higher their chances of making an Olympic team. Van Gogh placed 18th in the first stage of our race at the Energiewacht Tour, a windy, drizzly, 100-km slugfest against a field with multiple world champions competing. A very good placing, but not exactly an annihilation of her competitors. The next day, Van Gogh got tangled in a crash. It was at that point I got to experience racing with her.

Holland's most notorious competitor is wind, busting apart 200-person pelotons with hefty blows from the North Sea, sending riders into one another with shoulder bumps and handlebar entangling. I was a few rows behind Van

Gogh when she went down on the second day. The wind and the crash gapped us from the main field, segregating everyone behind the crash into small groups now chasing fervently to get back to the mothership of the peloton. Van Gogh's tumble wasn't a serious collision, and I looked back to see her remount her bike. A teammate of hers waited up the road, a smart tactical move to help one another get back to the peloton on such a windy day. I knew they'd come by my group and try to pass us, and I readied myself. As they passed, I jumped into the draft of Van Gogh.

For about 20 minutes, Van Gogh, her teammate, and I tried to bridge back to the main peloton. We rotated in a pace line—each of us taking turns drafting behind the other, to save energy and strength in the headwind. When Van Gogh rotated to the front and took her turn in the wind, she was strong, swift, and smooth. But she was not superhuman. She pulled just as hard as her teammate, and any other elite female cyclist I've raced with. Not more, not less. Equal.

Slogging away in the wind, my opinion of racing with transgendered athletes solidified as one of pride and respect. She was strong and determined, and to race with her in that moment also made me perform better. Her body wasn't a "he" or a "she" but an athlete doing what they do: competing to the best of their ability. Maybe my opinion will change if all of a sudden there are transgendered athletes taking over the podiums and dominating Olympic teams in all women's sports. But last time I checked, there weren't thousands of men rushing into surgery so they could compete with female athletes. Fifty years ago, transgender athletes weren't even in the mix—at least not publicly. Now they are. Such is the education of sport, ever evolving, asking us to do the same.

Drafting off Van Gogh, I thought of something else, too. The human element of all this transgender fuss. (Actually, I probably thought of it later as I don't think much on a bike. I only suffer, and that takes up most of my brain cells.) The opinions of other riders, coaches, managers, and race directors...surely not all are supportive of a transgendered female cyclist. It can't be easy for Van Gogh, having enemies or less-than-enthused people surround you in the middle of a peloton of 200 riders, where a quick elbow, intentional swerve, or shove is all it takes to send a certain message. Or worse, take out a rider at high speeds. I can only imagine Van Gogh's not had an easy transition into the ranks of pro cycling. But regardless of gender, an athlete is an athlete, and Natalie Van Gogh is a person who loves her sport. A person who loves to compete. A person who had to undergo something most of us don't—a surgical operation on the outside to be who you are on the inside. Gender aside, there is something we can all relate to about being human—being oneself is both the hardest and the easiest thing in the world. I applaud Van Gogh for sticking it out in cycling, for being herself.

Natalie shares her name with another famous Van Gogh—Vincent—who said of his own life journey, "I'm seeking, I am striving, I am in it with all my heart." So, too, is every great athlete, regardless of gender and sport. As our chase group battled to catch back on to the peloton, I could see the effort, intensity, and drive Natalie put into each pedal stroke. She was fatigued, relentless, and determined, just like the rest of us. In that seeking and striving moment of sport, she wasn't a man or a woman or a transgendered person. She was a competitor and an athlete and a bike racer. She was in it with all her heart.

THE GUY IN YELLOW
December 2013

"WHAT DO YOU THINK OF LANCE ARMSTRONG?"

No modern-day cyclist has gone a month without fielding this question from curious fans, skeptics, and most often outsiders of the sport. As a cyclist and a journalist, I've been asked countless times—not just since Armstrong made his infamous confession of taking performance-enhancing drugs, but for years beforehand as people speculated about his cleanliness. Controversy is always multi-faceted, and so I never have a single answer. I have four.

As a journalist, I'm exhausted by the constant Armstrong coverage and feel as most do—that more attention should be paid to other deserving athletes within cycling. (That's the easy one.)

As a cyclist, I'm just plain sad about the whole darn thing.

As a *female* cyclist, it is a struggle to constantly read how "cycling" is overcome with cheating and misconduct, rather than "men's cycling." While women's cycling has its issues, we don't share the same dark cloud of doping to the extent the men's field does. Perhaps, however, the silver lining in the Armstrong debacle is the opportunity he has inadvertently given the women's side of the sport. Maybe now there is an opening for our peloton to slip into

56

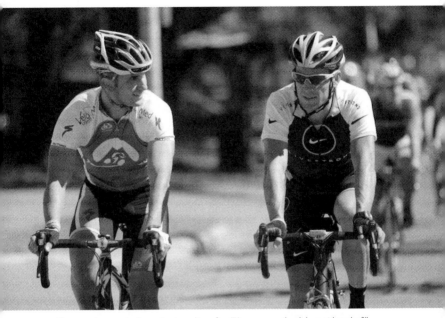

The secondmost-asked question in cycling after "How many miles did you ride today?" is—and might always be—"What do you think of Lance Armstrong?"

the limelight, to restore the faith of cycling fans, to shine a light on the unsung members of our athletic tribe. Perhaps the subtle, unintended gift of opportunity is something all fallen idols leave in their wake.

The fourth perspective is a little more complicated, caught somewhere in the quagmire of compassion and disappointment, camaraderie and disillusionment. What do I think of Lance Armstrong, not from the perspective of an athlete or journalist, but as a person?

There is a photograph of Armstrong on our wall, across from where I type these words. Actually, there are two pictures. One is a black and white glossy of Armstrong after his 2006 Tour de France victory, on which he's written, "To Colleen: Hang in there and LiveStrong!" Colleen was my husband's first wife.

The other photo is of my husband, George, riding alongside Armstrong in Austin, Texas, two weeks after Colleen passed away from breast cancer at age 31. The photo is in color, with the deep turquoise of my husband's cycling kit and the bold yellow of the Tour de France champion's helmet catching the sun in brilliant, vivacious tones. Lance is chatting with George. They are both smiling. Two guys on bikes, having a conversation about life, captured by a camera that for one moment of reprieve shows no inkling of the death and grief surrounding a young widower. When I look at that photo of Lance, I don't see a seven-time Tour de France champion. Nor do I see a man stripped of those titles. Or a man embattled in a web of lies and litigation. I see a guy wearing a yellow helmet, talking to a dude in a blue jersey who just lost his wife, and this yellow guy has somehow made this blue man smile.

While the world clamors to categorize Armstrong as a liar, a cheat, a bully, and a bad, bad man, in our household Lance Armstrong is still a human being. His photo remains where it is, hanging among other snapshots of things and people and places we take pride in remembering. Two guys on bikes, mid-conversation, smiling—I can find no ill will or harsh words to bestow upon someone who helped bring peace and joy to another in his time of greatest need.

We forget this too easily in the media, that winners and losers and cheaters and suspects are also, at their core, human beings who messed up. It is not difficult to rip apart those who have done wrong, or likewise to elevate others to the rank of hero too easily, especially on the vicious playgrounds of social media. I see Lance Supporters and Lance Haters launch wicked tirades at one another, and at Armstrong directly. I'm not of the opinion we should forgive and forget those who wreak havoc on the sports we love. Armstrong did wrong and caused severe damage, and it is good that we don't settle for such misconduct. Yet if the Armstrong situation brings about the necessary change we need in cycling, then perhaps there is a victory to be seen in this overwhelming dark cloud of drugs, dishonesty, and sport. It's a complicated condition to judge people who make cavernous mistakes.

Perhaps the Armstrong predicament touches a nerve in most of us because it confronts us with a deep psychological question: What do we make of people who commit acts both good and bad? Once a person steps out of the realm of such classification, it presents a confusing quandary. Do we continue to love what Armstrong has done for cancer patients and research, or do we solely focus on the destruction and deceit he's brought to cycling and fair play—is it even possible we can feel both, or are we contradicting and compromising ourselves in doing so? Maybe instead of asking what we think of Armstrong, it might serve us better to ask *how* we should think of Lance Armstrong. *How* provides a few more options, inviting us to consider not just his actions but our own boundaries of right and wrong, good and evil. *How* asks us to take a look at ourselves when considering the judgment of others. Armstrong will undoubtedly remain many things to many people: liar, hero, cheat, champion, ass, Olympian, loser, winner, a guy wearing yellow in a charity ride. However the classifications vary, somewhere among the choices and titles I hope "flawed human being" remains a quiet contender.

THE WATTIES
September 2011

IN SEPTEMBER 2011, *Bicycling Magazine* came out with a poll asking, "Who's the hottest female cyclist?" Five racers' photos were included. None of them pictured a cyclist in the heat of competition; most of the photos were glamour shots, and all of the cyclists are inarguably beautiful, wonderful women. Now, I'm not going to start preaching about sexism and equality and blah, blah, blah—I'm actually fine with this kind of hottie list coming from the likes of *Maxim, FHM,* or even *People*. That's what those publications do, and ranking physical beauty is their thing. But you know what else they do? Those magazines also *write* about the women in those photos.

Bicycling Magazine, however, a supposed "friend" in helping to promote women in sport, rarely gives professional (or amateur) female cycling any coverage at all. Three of the women in *Bicycling*'s hottie poll—Britain's Victoria Pendleton, the U.S.'s Dotsie Bausch, and Sweden's Emilia Fahlin—are so much more than beautiful faces. They are an Olympian, a world-record setter, and a national champion, respectively. But who would know that? From race results to training features to personal profiles, very little of *Bicycling Magazine*'s content is about women.

If *Bicycling*'s hottie list was one of many features on

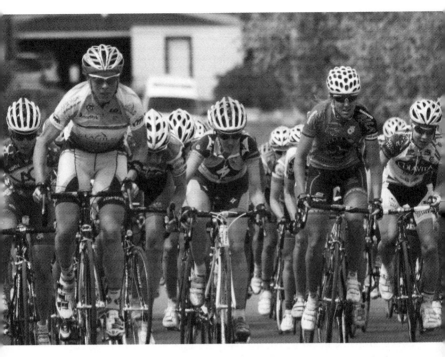

Watt: a unit of power. Cyclists use wattage to determine their power capacity. Hot: Yes, they are. (Nippy Feldhake III)

females, that would be one thing. But it's not. So the hottie list is just a tad insulting when it's the only time *Bicycling* pays attention to the fantastic females of the sport. And honestly, it makes the magazine look just plain silly. *Bicycling Magazine* rating female pro cyclists on their looks is like *Entertainment Weekly* grading opera performances.

Either stick to what you know, *Bicycling*—mass-market male clothing and high-end bikes for triple-chain-ring weekend warriors—or start covering women regularly and knowledgeably. Start measuring talent by watts, not hots.

If you're going to rank a female athlete, here's the right way to do it:

Announcing, in no particular order, the first-ever 10 Super Female Watties of Road Cycling where physical power *is* beauty. Vote for a winner if you must, but I think these top 10 (plus three) are all equally awesome.

Jeannie "Did you call me old? I can't hear you way back there" Longo (FRA)

Longo has the winningest record in the history of cycling—male or female. She's now 52 and still ruling the game. People who scroll through Longo's list of national, world, and Olympic titles usually get carpal tunnel syndrome before they're done.

Kristin "Mama's gonna knock you out" Armstrong (USA)

Armstrong won gold in the time trial at the Beijing Games. She retired, had a baby, and recently unretired for a shot at the 2012 Olympics. Don't call it a comeback—she's been here for years.

Giorgia "The real Italian Stallion" Bronzini (ITA)

Reigning world road race champion Bronzini is a force to be reckoned with. A deadly sprint and unwavering toughness make her one of the best competitors on the pro circuit. She's the cyclist you'd least like to meet in a dark alley and most want to have on your team.

Greta "It's my legs you should worry about" Neimanas (USA)

Neimanas is an amazing cyclist. A 2008 U.S. Paralympic Team member and multiple medalist in world and national events, Neimanas is also a member of the stellar pro team Peanut Butter & Co. TWENTY12, competing regularly against all classifications of cyclists. Competitors rarely notice Neimanas has only one arm. After all, it's her powerful legs they need to worry about. This athlete should be on every top-10 list of badass women in sports.

Marianne "Nice girls come in first" Vos (NED)

Vos has gold medals and world titles all over the place, but you'd never guess it. Humble, gracious, ego-free, and approachable, Vos has the ability to domestique for her team-mates as well as dominate as a champion. She is cycling's model of how a champion pro athlete should behave.

Coryn "Most people have socks older than me" Rivera (USA)

Rivera, who recently turned 18, has already won 32 U.S. national championship gold medals in road, track, and cyclocross racing disciplines. She is the most decorated junior cyclist in America, male or female. Watching her rise through cycling (and the peloton) is a terrific experience.

Clara "Asphalt, ice...whatever. Your choice. I'll destroy you on either" Hughes (CAN)

Hughes is shooting for her sixth Olympic Games in 2012. Even more impressive is the fact she's an Olympian in two sports—cycling and speedskating—with six Olympic medals to date (four bronze, one silver, one gold). This year, Hughes is capturing nearly every time-trial title en route to London. Topping it all off, she's a happy person with a great smile. Even when destroying her competition.

Amber "I'm just a little thing…and I will rip your legs off with my teeth" Neben (USA)

Neben is all of 5'3" and hardly over 100 lbs., resembling a coxswain more than a cyclist. But don't let her size fool you. Neben is the 2009 world champion in the time trial and an Olympian to boot. Tough as nails, Neben has beaten spinal meningitis and cancer, proving so far that nothing can keep her down. With her six wins and a multitude of podium placings in 2011, we're betting nothing ever will.

Jessica "If you build it, they will come" Phillips (USA)

Phillips has two major titles under her belt, a 2002 road-racing national championship and 2009 time-trial title. She could have stopped there, but in 2011 Phillips went on to a more impressive feat: organizing a top-level pro race for women in Colorado. When she heard the men's U.S. Pro Cycling Challenge didn't have a women's event, she watted up and made one happen in the Aspen/Snowmass Women's Pro Stage Race. One small step for women, one giant step for cyclingkind. Thank you, Jessica.

Evelyn "I can analyze your stock portfolio between intervals" Stevens (USA)

In 2009, Stevens went from Wall Street analyst to pro bike racer in just more than a year, garnering a world team spot and a 2011 national championship in her newbie debut.

And here is a special Watties nod to three of the hotties *Bicycling* didn't do justice to:

Emilia "I'm really pretty...clueless as to why *Bicycling* failed to mention I also kick ass" Fahlin (SWE)

Twenty-two-year-old Swedish sprinter Fahlin has already been the national champion on the road and in the time trial. The cycling world is Fahlin's oyster, and a long career awaits this terrific athlete.

Dotsie "Yes, I'm a model...a role model" Bausch (USA)

Bausch is a six-time U.S. national champion, two-time Pan Am champion, and part of a team pursuit world-record-breaking team. Off the bike, she's a cycling coach and a model who touts the message of wellness for women everywhere. Now that's what we call an all-around role model.

Victoria "Secret ain't half as sexy as my world-dominating quads" Pendleton (GBR)

Pendleton is a British, Olympic, and world track champion who's been a force since 1999 and is a member of the superhuman Team Sky. Still going strong, Pendleton is a main contender on the track for London 2012. *Bicycling* polled her for being hot, but like every other woman on this list, Pendleton should be celebrated for her watts—of which she generates many.

So go ahead and keep your hottie list, *Bicycling*. While the world will continue to rank women on looks, magazines will continue to poll athletes on their faces instead of feats, and female athletes will continue to struggle for equality, we can change one thing—female athletes can make our own lists, ranks, and polls of what really matters, and we can live by those standards until the rest of the world catches up.

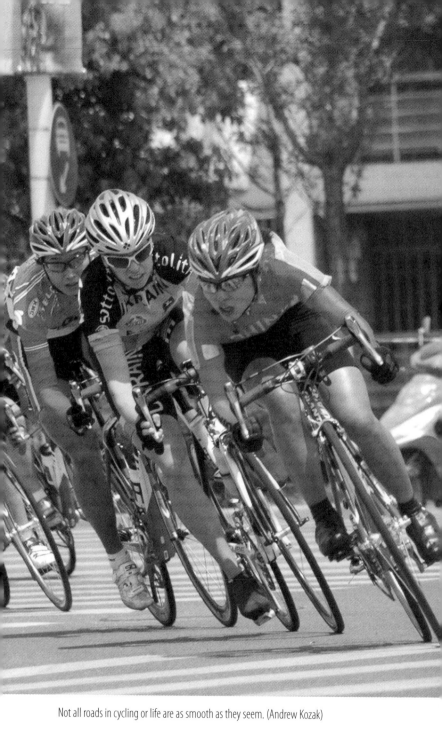

Not all roads in cycling or life are as smooth as they seem. (Andrew Kozak)

PART II:
ROUGH ROAD

There are times in every journey where the path navigates a fine line between devastation, ridiculousness, and patience. The most infuriating obstacles on my road through the cycling world often came with an edge of humor, while the emotional moments sometimes just needed room to breathe. How is it possible we live in a world where bicycles are charged $525 at an airport, where there is no lunch at world championships, and where a bicycle hanging on a wall means so much more than a bicycle hanging on wall? Tears, laughter, and compassion seemed interchangeable, and change itself became a quiet yet powerful road slowly winding its way through my words.

MAPS
May 2011

I'M FLYING INTO MEDELLIN, Colombia, site of the 2011 Pan American Cycling Championships, and the woman seated next to me is Colombian. She mentions how everyone in her country loves athletes, how there are so many local bike clubs, and she begins to passionately describe nearby cycling routes as her hands enthusiastically gesticulate steep climbs and twisting roads. "Here," she says. "Let me draw you a map."

On the back of an airline napkin, she draws hills that look disproportionally large—nearly cascading off the ridge of the napkin—and I stifle a giggle at her penned exaggerations. We are flying in at night, so it isn't until morning that I see her drawing is frighteningly accurate. When we deplane, she wishes me luck in my time trial and road race.

Perhaps more than in most sports, luck is a necessity for cyclists. Preparation, hard work, and mental toughness are key, but no amount of training can save a rider from flat tires, unseen potholes, group crashes, or whether or not a baggage handler ultimately decides to put one's bike on the plane.

In fact, the cardinal rule of competitive cycling is that there's rarely a perfect race, especially when competing abroad. During the last four years, I've conditioned myself

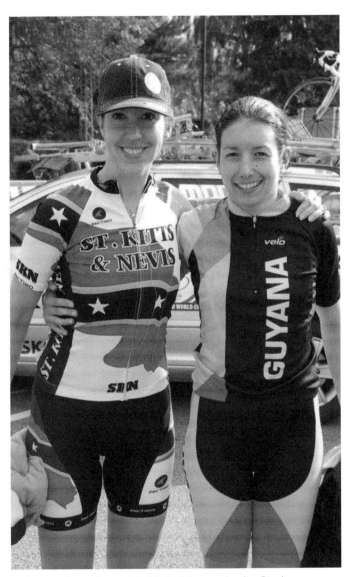

Not knowing where you're going is half the battle in women's cycling. Friends (and maps) are key. Here I am with fellow small-nation racer Claire Fraser-Green of Guyana. (Shaun Green)

to expect the unexpected. Sometimes luck—good or bad—is just another synonym for adventure. Since adopting this philosophy, every trip's been virtually easy. Like this one to Colombia:

The hotel doesn't have running water? Ok, so I'll stink for a few days.

No one here speaks English? Que interesada!

Can't identify the meat in my free athlete's dinner? Tastes like pollo!

My debit card's been stolen! I can still get a combo on the dollar menu.

We have to race at 6,500 feet? It's nice to have pretty scenery while dying.

The bus transporting us to the race venue is an hour late and I only have 15 minutes to warm up before the time trial, which is vital to my Olympic quest? Fear of missing your start is, in fact, the most effective way to quickly raise one's heart rate.

Luck, adventure—it's all the same. So you can imagine my surprise when my time trial not only went off without a hitch, but I actually had a really good race. I finished a solid 12th and covered the 20-km course at altitude—which I refer to as owwtitude—in 28:45. The upside was that places No. 6 through 12 were only separated by 32 seconds. I closed the gap on many competitors who were far ahead of me in previous years. Personal improvement has occurred, and there is now a chance I'll be invited to the quadrennial Pan American Games in Mexico this October. That could lead to an Olympic berth.

So, all things considered, not being able to shower for a couple days isn't such a bad trade-off.

As for the road race, that's where my luck ran out. Or, more accurately, wooshed out. Less than 10 kilometers into the 96-km race, a giant South American pothole assaulted my rear wheel and deflated my chances of staying in the peloton.

Despite getting a wheel change from the support car, the lost time and difficult new gearing for a very hilly course (I was given a wheel with an 11x21 cassette, for all you cycling nerds) left me with two options: quit, or keep riding and finish the race despite any chance of getting back to the peloton. I'm not one for quitting, especially when the time, energy, money, and mental fortitude it took to get to Colombia totals a hefty price. Flats happen—that's part of bike racing. But quitting is always a choice.

I've learned time and again that when mapping out dreams and goals in cycling, it's usually best to use pencil instead of pen.

While I didn't get any Olympic points here in Colombia, this is the closest I have come yet. Doors have been opened and fitness has been elevated. More important, personal growth has occurred.

Here in South America, I met a new rider from Guyana, Claire Fraser. She is also on her own quest to qualify for the Games and was disappointed when her results in the time trial and road race did not turn out as she'd hoped.

I told her what I'd learned from my own Olympic quest—luck, hard work, pencil usage, and simply paying your dues in terms of experience...and how I, too, came in nearly last at my first Pan Am Championships.

"It's just frustrating when races don't go according to your plan," Fraser said. That's when I told her about perseverance and how following that path is the best way to get anywhere.

"Here," I said. "Let me draw you a map."

LUNCH AND OTHER OBSTACLES
December 2011

LAST WEEK IN COPENHAGEN, Denmark, at the 2011 Road World Championships in cycling, Fabian Cancellara, a four-time world champion, made a costly error in navigating a tight turn in the time trial.

While Cancellara didn't crash after overshooting the tricky corner, he had to come to a dead stop to avoid doing so, proving that the course was insanely difficult at high speeds. There were slick cobblestones, narrow corners, small European streets, rainy weather, nasty headwinds, and ruthless competitors.

"What about for you?" asked a friend, who had seen Cancellara's corner and wondered how someone with, um, slightly lesser skill had fared on such a course. I, too, was at the world championships, competing for the fourth time. "What was the toughest part of racing worlds?" I thought it over carefully.

"Lunch," I said. Sometimes the hardest part about going after an Olympic dream has nothing to do with sports.

Over the past four years of chasing my Olympic qualification dream, I've learned that racing is less than half the battle. It's about the little things that aren't so apparent. Because I race for a nation unable to support its cyclists financially (I have dual citizenship with St. Kitts and Nevis),

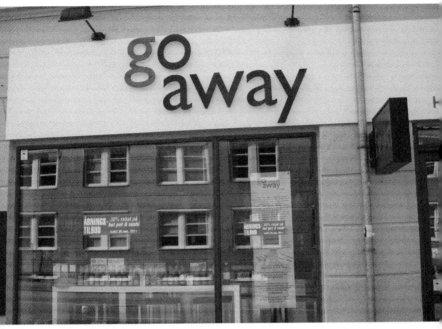

As if it isn't hard enough to find lunch abroad, it doesn't help when restaurants in Denmark miss the mark on translation.

the logistics leading up to the races are usually harder than any cobblestone corner. Getting there is the first step.

Flying for 16 hours with two bikes, having no budget for a hotel or rental car, and hoping the male homestay I'd found through Facebook wasn't a serial killer made up most of my world championships concerns. (It's cool—Jens used smiley face icons when we communicated via email, so I knew he'd be a good person.) Anyway, while most of my competitors spend their prerace routine navigating a mental and physical route to victory, I ruminate on the odds of being within walking distance of a grocery store. After all, you can't win a time trial if you can't score lunch first.

Sure, the fully funded teams have it easier. Things like food, beds, and transportation are provided. There are team mechanics, doctors, massage therapists, coaches, and lunch shoppers/makers on hand to allow the athletes to focus solely on the sport. My journey is a little different, but when my bike is creaky, my solo-ness gets tricky, and the grocery store closes earlier than expected, I just have to remember one thing: I'm lucky to be here. Finishing 44th might not come with a medal, but it always awards perspective.

Lucky for me, Denmark turned out to be a good trip. My homestay was fantastic. I could walk to the grocery store and ride my bike to the time trial course. I needed help with other logistics, but I managed. And the cobblestone corners turned out to be my friend. Despite my seemingly far-away-from-winning 44th place in the time trial, my time and my speed average (just over 25 mph for a technical 27K course) were my best to date, and I'm only a couple minutes away from the top 20. I've improved, and the Olympic dream is still alive.

But my friend's question about the "toughest part" got me thinking. There's a lot about the world championships that people probably don't realize, especially from the non-podium perspective. Television captures the winners but not so much what it's like behind the scenes and for smaller nations. So here's a list of the top eight largely unknown facts about the world championships of cycling, as experienced by a non-famous competitor.

1. Strange men ask me for my clothing.

Occasionally, security will let cycling fans wander

through the warm-up tents. Most are European men who collect weird things. They often ask me for a St. Kitts and Nevis team jersey, hat, gloves, etc. I explain that there are no extras, that I have to buy my own team uniform. They linger, waiting for me to change my mind. The security man does not come over. He is busy smoking. I retreat to my backup plan and start my "strange facial tic" routine. Very soon they leave me alone.

2. The time trial warm-up tent is like an athletic version of a suspect interrogation room.

Wealthy men's cycling teams have extravagant team buses to keep athletes safe and warm during warm-up time. But for most women's national teams traveling half-way around the globe to get to worlds, we get a chair and a table, usually under a weather-challenged 8' x 8' tent. They look like 50 little suspect interrogation rooms. Mind you, I'm quite grateful for this. Having the use of a table and chair is a step up for my unranked federation.

3. Team cars are for…teams.

While the major teams in women's cycling are given a car to follow the peloton with spare wheels and bikes, the UWFs (unknown women federations of pro cycling)—nations with just one or two riders—are herded into shared cars. That means the car may or may not stop if you have an emergency, depending on if you're more or less important than your fellow nation. Car sharing at worlds is like the start of a bad joke. *A Croatian, a Syrian, and a tropical islander are in the back seat of a Skoda...*

4. The UCI is now regulating pelvic bones.

There are all sorts of inane rules in cycling, among them the positioning of time trial bikes. The bikes have to weigh so much, measure that much, have this or that angle. Right before the start of the time trial, a stodgy man in a business suit decrees the proper angle of every cyclist's saddle by placing a level on it. Despite the fact that bicycles are built so the saddle can be tilted slightly up or down to fit the rider's pelvis dimensions, the UCI has now declared that a saddle must be perfectly level. If it's not, the rider must "fix" the bike to this man's standards, often resulting in a different riding position and a fair amount of inner angst. This new rule was created to uphold the UCI's creed on technological advancement: "If it ain't broke, let me find my sledgehammer."

5. Unranked riders are sent to the back.

While every other race on the UCI calendar allows riders to place themselves at the start line in whatever fashion they choose, at world championships, the small nations and unranked riders are forced to let the more "important" athletes ahead of them at the start. Sure, the ranked countries have earned the right to be recognized, but if the emerging nations are kept at the back, perhaps they'll struggle longer. The upside is that at the back of the pack, there's lots of camera time on my backside. Okay, maybe that's not an upside.

6. The sound of one hand clapping is actually quite loud.

There are five identifiable species of world championship applause: Thunderous, Drunken, Sarcastic, the Mom Clap, and the Sound of One Hand Clapping. The first two are similar and are the best reward any athlete can receive for their effort and pain. The world championships draw large crowds of European cycling fans who often like to party during a race that lasts up to four hours.

Sarcastic clapping coming from the "fans" is often reserved for struggling riders. It's rather mean but luckily the rarest of the applause categories.

Sarcastic clapping is offset by the Mom Clap, which comes from the devoted people in the crowd who firmly believe that every rider needs encouragement. Strong, clear, loud, and rhythmic, the Mom Clap is often accompanies by phrases like, "You're almost there," "You can win this," and "Don't give up," despite the fact the athlete is often 10 minutes or more behind the leader.

The Sound of One Hand Clapping is the newest member of the applause family tree. Plastic hand-shaped toys that issue a *thwack-thwack-thwack* when shaken vigorously now offer an alternative for people too lazy to bring their own two hands together. Either way, it works. Cyclists at the front and the back of the peloton enjoy it greatly.

7. BYOTP

Even for the greatest cycling competitors at worlds, the Porta-Potties never have toilet paper.

8. We get by with a little help from our friends.

So, all in all, there's no free lunch for the smaller countries at the world champs, but there are people who help keep our heads off the platter. The Mexican team helped me out with a gearing issue and lent me some spare parts. The Shimano guy gave me a front wheel when mine developed a problem. The Guyanese team gave me a ride to the road course every day when they learned I could not afford a rental car. The lady in the supermarket, noticing I was foreign, pointed out I'd selected buttermilk in my failed attempt to find skim.

All of these moments were small battles that could have cost me the war had I not had some help during worlds. Next time a world championship race is on TV or maybe even in your town, watch and cheer on the best of the best. And maybe even bring a snack for the girls in the back, forever trying their best to get up to the front.

UNITED WE FALL
September 2009

A CYCLIST WALKS INTO an airport and goes to the United Airlines counter to check in.

The woman behind the desk says, "Where you going today?"

The cyclist says, "Switzerland."

The woman behind the desk says, "How many bags?"

The cyclist says, "One."

The woman behind the desk says, "That'll be $525 for the bag, please."

The cyclist says, "Wait…this isn't a joke?"

The woman behind the desk says, "No."

The cyclist then understands that United Airlines is the Devil.

And so began my trip to the 2009 world championships in cycling, where I was wallet-raped by United Airlines in broad daylight in the middle of the Phoenix airport. While this might seem like an essay on the complaints of modern-day baggage robbery, it is actually a glimpse behind the iron curtain of how the *other* pro athletes—as in, the not-yet-famous-but-hoping-to-get-there—make it or break it in their respective fields of dreams.

Lance Armstrong, for example, didn't need to worry about bike-baggage fees because the dude had his own jet.

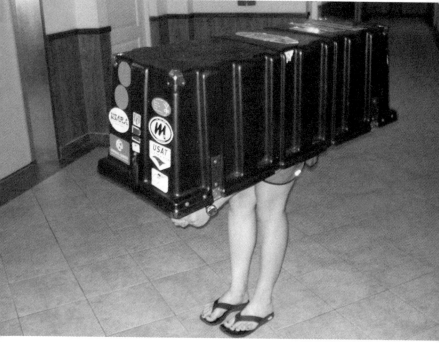

A bicycle suitcase. Also serves as a direct portal to airport hell.

I, on the other hand, race for a small country (St. Kitts and Nevis) that cannot offer sponsorship or financial assistance to help get me to races. So baggage fees and travel come out of my pocket. That's okay. That's how it goes in sports. I don't want a medal or a cookie or a pat on the back for my efforts. What I do want is fair play. United, it seems, is the worst opponent an Olympic hopeful could ask for.

Once upon a time, my bike flew to Europe for free on United. A couple of years later, $525 *one way*. First, a disclaimer: I am very, very, very poor at all things mathematical. If there is a clinical level of mental ineptitude in math, then I possess that diagnosis. At the very least, I can add and subtract most numbers with three digits or less but I do have to use my fingers and/or talk out loud while problem solving. Now, back to the Devil.

In front of me, a family of five (two adults and three young children) checked the allotted two bags per person onto their international flight. The parents obviously enjoyed their shopping trip to the United States, as they had a total of 10 bags, each of which weighed 50 pounds. They were using their three children as luggage mules, but according to United this is not a problem. The family was not charged any baggage fees. I even watched as one bag weighed in at 52 pounds, but the ticket agent sighed and said, "Well, okay, I'll let it go for this one." So tell me, United, how a 5-year-old can legally check two bags totaling 100 pounds for free, but a grown woman gets charged $525 for one box? Something doesn't add up.

But wait, there's more!

I do understand there is a fee for overweight bags these days. Fifty dollars is the norm, it seems. Bikes sometimes get charged $150. Annoying, but I'll pay it. But when the woman at the ticket counter charged me $175 for the bike then added the $350 overweight charge, I was outraged but also confused. If the bike fee is supposed to incorporate the bulky, large, heavy charge, then why was I being charged twice? She cleared it up by saying, "There is nothing I can do."

I asked for her supervisor. That's when things got nasty.

Supervisor Devil came over and said there was nothing *she* could do. I pointed out the luggage-mule-children before me, and she said, "Those people have normal bags. You are not normal."

Well, my un-normalcy is not news to me, but being out-right insulted by a United rep was definitely new ground. Only family and friends have the right to un-normalize me. Not strangers! The ticket lady then said, "Can you take anything out of the box to make it lighter?"

Then things got just plain stupid. Inside my bike box were two bike frames and the little bag that holds their dis-assembled components (saddles, pedals, etc). I told her I could take out the little bag and put it in my carry-on, but what difference would that make? Isn't it all going on the same plane? Again, my math skills are weak, but I felt my logic was adding up.

The ticket woman shook her head and said, "There is nothing I can do." She then added, "You have 10 minutes to check your bag, or it won't get on the flight." So there I was. I had to pay the $525 or my bikes wouldn't make it to worlds and I wouldn't get to race. I forked over the money.

A moment of clarification for those wondering, "Hey, dumbass, why didn't you ship your bikes by UPS or rent a bike in Switzerland?" Good questions but improbable solutions. If I ship my bikes (time trial and road) to Europe, I am left without my bikes for two weeks prior to the most impor-tant race of the year. This would be the equivalent of asking a swimmer to stay out of the pool two weeks leading up to the Olympics. Renting a bike, similarly, would be like asking a baseball player to use someone else's glove during the World Series or a marathoner to wear someone else's shoes. Or maybe like asking the Devil to use someone else's pitchfork to spear some poor soul into air-travel hell. Just doesn't work.

Destitute and dispirited, I made my way to the terminal. A man approached me. He observed my ticket-counter esca-pades and introduced himself as an elite wrestling coach, also traveling to a competition in Europe. He told me he'd checked seven bags for his athletes and was not charged a penny because United supports his Olympic-hopeful team. I went back to the counter and found the supervisor. I told her that I, too, am an Olympic hopeful for 2012.

"Do you have a coupon?" she asked. "A voucher?"

"I need a voucher for hope?"

"Yes, you do for United."

"Please, ma'am. I'm representing a country at the world championships."

"There's nothing I can do."

I got on the plane, broke in wallet and spirit, and spent the next 12 hours wondering what happened to customer service, mourning the death of common sense, and nearly crying tears of laughter over the fact that United sponsors the charity Feeding America but won't give its 250 passengers a free sandwich.

When I got to Switzerland, I came in 37th in the stacked field at the world championships. It was a good day. Then I got charged $220 for the bike box on the way home. At a total of $745, the cost for my bike to race at worlds actually exceeded that of my plane ticket. So goes a week in the life of an Olympic-hopeful cyclist.

Now, I may be pitiful at math, but I'm pretty sure my real problem with United's equation lay in the fact that not all are considered equal. I don't know much about devilish corporate policy, hellish baggage monopolies, or why common sense went belly-up, but I do know that one girl with a bike and a dream, one wrestling coach with magical vouchers, and one 5-year-old with bags that outweigh him need to be treated as equal players in the consumer game. I also really want to return to my career as a sports journalist and not spend any more time attempting to reach United's customer service department (so far the count is three disconnected, half-hour calls in the past six hours). Hopefully United will come around and fix this issue. Until then I'm afraid my new motto is: United we fall, divided I...wait, division. That's the one with the little line and two dots, right?

After weeks of calling United, and sending extensive emails to their corporate office, the airline issued me a voucher for $500 good toward a future United flight. I used the refund to bring my husband to my next race. I poked holes in the bike box so he could breathe.

THE PINARELLO
December 2010

HANGING FROM INDIVIDUAL hooks along a wall in our garage, our eight bicycles dangle from their front wheels, pedals angled to accommodate each other in synchronicity, a motionless kick line of carbon fiber Rockettes. My husband and I are competitive cyclists. I race professionally, George races at the very competitive amateur level known as Category 3.[3] George is a self-proclaimed gear junkie, deeply in love with the mechanics and components of finely crafted bicycles. He happily spends hours in his man cave, doting on his two wheeled possessions, tending to filthy chains with gentle Q-tips, wiping drips of sticky endurance drinks hard-crusted along the top tube with loving care and Simple Green, while rags of old race T-shirts hang staunchly throughout his workstation, caked with the evidence of his pride in cleanliness. I, on the other hand, feel no pull toward the technical element of cycling. I am happy if my wheels are round and my frame is light enough to keep up with my competition. Perhaps it is largely a female trait, but I'm simply not as keen to spend my free time in

---

3 In USA Cycling regulations, cyclists compete in categories based on experience, "catting up" from level to level based on wins, rankings, and points. Category 5 is beginner cyclist, Category 1 is professional-level cyclist.

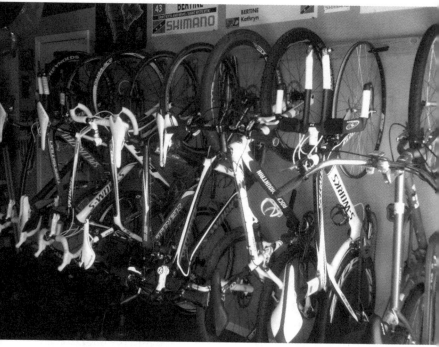

Bikes lie in wait in a cyclists' garage.

the garage. Though I admit, the wall of bikes is lovely in formation.

Three of the bikes in the garage are mine—road, time trial, and commuter. Four are George's—two road, one time trial, one mountain bike. The eighth bike belonged to Colleen, my husband's first wife who passed away from cancer. She rode a small Pinarello road bike, black carbon with blue and white paint adorning the high-end frame. From one of the middle hooks, the bike dangles wheel-less from the triangular crux of the rear chain-stay. The Pinarello's empty front fork rests against the garage wall. The wheels have been reassigned to one of the other bikes, leaving the Pinarello to hang at an awkward angle, half of itself. The handlebar tape is scuffed and the rubber brake hood is slightly ripped after a friend borrowed the bike for a local race and went down in a troublesome corner. Scratched, too, is the paint near the rear derailleur. The wounds are superficial; the bike is still in fine condition. And yet it pains me to look at the Pinarello on a daily basis, saddens me to my core every time I head into the garage. To see something so reminiscent of life, something in itself the very nature of forward movement, something once raced and ridden with the muscles and determination of a life at full momentum, now dismantled and left to stillness…this weighs on me until I silently agree to dissect the emotion.

We have some things that belonged to Colleen, though we have given many away. The most personal items, like clothing and jewelry and family photographs, were given to her parents. George keeps a small satchel with their wedding rings and a shoebox of photographs. Helmets and jerseys and law school books went to friends who could use them. In our new home, George and I merged the furniture of our past places into a new one. The dining table, the downstairs sofa, the guest bedroom furniture, and some paintings come from the life George shared with Colleen. Our bedroom, office desk, and upstairs sofa come from my old condo. Around the house, a mirror and a giraffe statue and kitchen knickknacks that were once Colleen's now mingle with picture frames and photo albums and book case that are mine. Not once has the sight of something she owned given me a negative feeling or brought strange associations to the forefront of my mind. Instead, I find peace in their existence—proof that positive memories prevail in the long run, that tangible reminders of the past can coexist with the present. Even in death, her notes scrawled in a cookbook or her dog-eared novels intermingled in our bookshelf continue to offer something to our daily life that George and I have constructed in this second chapter of marriage.

But the bicycle hanging there in the garage, trapped in stillness, breaks my heart. The saddle is the hardest part. I can see the wear and tear, the rubbed-away lettering of the brand name, the faded white leather creased with age and use, and the slightest bend from where her weight rested upon it. The handlebar tape is worn down where her gloved hands gripped the bars. Strange are the things we render personal. This is not her hairbrush or her eyeglasses or a handwritten letter but a conglomeration of metal and carbon and leather…all angled to fit the dimensions of a specific body that no longer exists. But I suppose I don't see a bicycle, after all. I see a racehorse without its rider, a shoe without its runner, a podium without its victor. I see one thing that needs another to make it whole. It is the motionlessness that makes me ache when I see her bike.

I want the bicycle to be used. I want to set it free as though it were a trapped bird, wheels spinning like wings with a new breath of wind. I want George to send it to Colleen's cousin up in Washington state, a young girl who has taken a shine to triathlon. I want, I want, I want. But George is not ready to send the bicycle away. It will take him a year and a half to get to the point where he can let it go. In the meantime, there are countless guests who, upon getting a tour of George's cycling man cave, ask us which bikes belong to whom…then navigate a gentle awkwardness when we get to Colleen's. It will take a year and a half of small arguments, as my offer to put new handlebar tape on her bike so at least it doesn't look so disheveled is met with a gruff, "I'll do it," which doesn't get done. I must remember there is much more on that eighth garage hook than I can see. This is not my road to travel; this is neither my journey nor my bicycle. It will take time for George to take something so tangible and switch it over to the realm of memory. But once there, among his private recollections, I believe the Pinarello will not live on a hook in a garage. It will race brilliantly down long forgotten roads with Colleen in the saddle, thriving and vibrant, navigating her private, invisible route between worlds past and present.

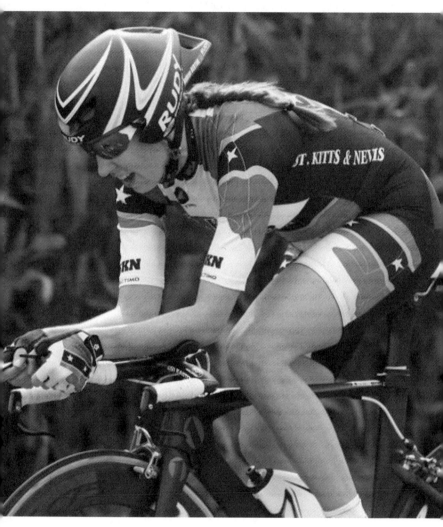

On the time trial course at the world championships, Limburg 2012. No stopping allowed.
(Danielle Moonen)

PART III:
NO STOPPING

Throughout my goal to turn professional and my second Olympic quest, I found inspiration and passion in the beauty of not stopping, no matter how high the odds were stacked. There were times I struggled to believe in myself, and during those moments I did what all humans do: I wavered and wondered and what-if'd whether or not the journey was worth it. Then I did that other thing that human bodies were built to do: keep going.

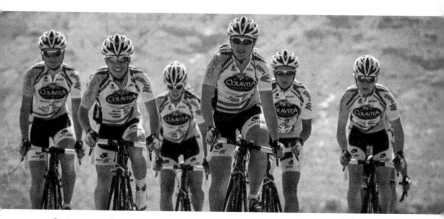

Getting on a professional team is the ultimate goal of most female racers. Five straight years of resume rejection, not so much. (Jonathan Devich/epicimages.us)

THE CALL UP
March 2012

IN FEBRUARY 2007, I entered my first bike race, the Usery Pass Omnium in Arizona. The first stage was a time trial that took less than 20 minutes but provided plenty of time for me to make four awesome rookie mistakes:

- I pinned on my race numbers upside down.
- I forgot to fill my water bottle.
- I didn't tighten down my clip-on aerobars, one of which began to dangle in the wind.
- I blocked the finish line by standing around, talking to a friend, incurring screams from the race director (through a megaphone) to get out of the way.

The race director and his militant microphone kept addressing me by number, 252.

"Get off the course, 252!"

I checked my backward, upside-down, block-print number. As far as I knew, I was 525 and very glad not to be 252. I didn't figure it out until he angrily stormed toward me. To this day, I can recall him walking away, shaking his head in frustration and mumbling something less than complimentary about Category 4 beginner riders.

Nine months later, after an intense gestation of carrying ESPN's Olympic-qualification-dream-via-cycling-journalist, I raced myself into the pro-level rank of Category 1. The rank gave me eligibility to race with the pros at the highest level, but it didn't guarantee a professional team would ever sign me to its roster. While I had improved greatly in nine months, in many ways I was still an infant rookie. I was also 31 years old—not the most helpful age, as international cycling rules called for the majority of riders on a professional women's team to have a racing age of less than 28 years old. I was on the wrong side of that ridiculous age-discriminating bookend. Not to mention, my ESPN assignment had ended, and no longer was I paid to write about my training and racing. The real world of stability and normalcy called—loudly—but the dream of cycling myself onto a professional team countered with screeching ferocity. *I have never been nor do I want to be normal! I don't even know what that means!* All I knew was my journey with cycling was not finished. What began as a journalism project had typed its way into my soul, imbuing a new lead and a fresh contract. I didn't race for ESPN anymore; I raced for myself and for my own dreams. I was determined to be signed by a pro team.

In 2008, I sent résumés to the best teams in the United States—Webcor, ValueAct, Cheerwine, TiBCO, Aaron's, PROMAN, Colavita—listing my above-average results and metaphorically offering my internal organs for the chance to domestique or, in non-cycling terms, gut myself to help a teammate win.

I sent emails and letters and left voicemail messages. I heard crickets.

I raced on local Tucson-based teams or joined composite rosters as the St. Kitts and Nevis national champion. *Try again next year*, I whispered internally. In 2009, I sent résumés to all the aforementioned teams, plus the new ones, Team Type 1, LipSmacker, Veloforma, and Touchstone.

Again, crickets. (Crickets faintly snickering.)

Same thing for 2010. And 2011. I wasn't getting younger, but my body was getting stronger. I made a deal with myself that as long as I kept improving, there was no reason to stop stalking every pro team on the planet, no matter how many turned me down. Rejection never bothered me, and I don't really believe in failure, preferring to hold fast to the notion that even the most resounding "no" is better than the quietest "what if?" I can live with rejection and the misconception of failure, but I can't live with *not trying*. So I kept applying to pro teams and kept getting "no" or crickets. In the interim, I rode with some great regional teams, including Specialized-Missing Link and Trisports, but the goal of racing professionally continued to elude me.

In late 2011, I got a break. Almost. A new UCI Dutch team was forming, and the owner asked if I wanted to be part of it. Indeed I did, and I started a little happy dance around my desk during our Skype call. *My first pro contract, my first pro contract, happy, happy contract....* But less than a month later, financial woes hit the director and the team folded before it began. The crickets sent their chirpy condolences.

In 2012, I put the pro team dream on the back burner to concentrate on earning St. Kitts and Nevis a berth to the London Games. After missing the mark on gaining enough qualifying points to Beijing four years ago, I buckled down into my training and readjusted my sights on a new Olympic path. By this point, I was used to racing solo, anyway.

And then, one day in early 2012, an email surfaced. It was from John Profaci, the head of Colavita Forno D'Asolo, the highest-ranked U.S. women's professional cycling team on the NRC (national race calendar) circuit. The team was forced to shut its doors at the close of 2011 when a financial partner pulled out, but Profaci was still looking to rebuild his cycling empire.

"Could you help me?" Profaci asked, referring to the many details it takes to get a team off the ground—marketing, writing, editing, introductions, finding riders and partners, etc. I gave a resounding "yes," more than happy to help. After all, I thought, *If I can't be on a pro team, at least I can help one find sponsors.*

And then, after six years of crickets, Profaci said, "Will you ride for us?"

All too wary about the possibility of another new team's failure to launch, I squeaked out a gun-shy "yes" but saved the happy dance. Instead, I asked important questions. Namely, could I still go to my Olympic qualifiers? Yes. The new Colavita team would get a late start, and my international Olympic qualifiers (which end in May) would not interfere with the team's domestic race schedule. The team might even be able to go to a couple qualifiers, which would only help me. Well, okay then! John and I started laying the behind-the-scenes groundwork for the team to come to fruition.

On February 1, 2012, at age 36, I signed my first pro cycling contract, complete with my first professional happy dance. Five years had passed since that first bike race with the upside-down race numbers and that Category 4 beginner who had a professional cycling dream. I still make rookie mistakes, just not as many, and this time I can use my knowledge of what *not* to do to help younger riders on our team thrive. Looking back, here are four things I know now that I didn't know then:

1. Just because a dream doesn't adhere to our preferred timeline doesn't mean it won't come true.

2. Thirty-six isn't old, not for a woman in an endurance sport. Or for anything else.

3. Try, ask, and apply for everything you ever want in life. You may hear crickets.

4. In some countries, they eat crickets for breakfast. So keep trying.

WELCOME TO THE HOPE SHOW
May 2012

THE BIGGEST JUXTAPOSITION about reaching the Olympics is it requires both Everyone and No One to get there.

First, there's the Everyone: the mechanics at Fair Wheel Bikes who keep my machine working; the home stays, race directors, and foreign team managers who helped me while abroad; and the emotional strength supplied by my husband and friends at my highest and lowest points. There is no way I could complete this Olympic quest on my own.

And yet, there's No One. Despite the fact I'm now fortunate enough to be on a professional team, my team does not necessarily go to the same races I need to attend for Olympic qualification points. For many events, I'm on my own. When I'm on the start line of a race, it's just my bike and me. As the lone female cyclist for St. Kitts and Nevis, I haven't had a team of riders to work with in Olympic qualification races. No one is there to protect me from the wind, lead me out in sprints, fetch water bottles from the team car (seeing as there is no team car), or strategize about how best to win.

Yet I can't complain at all; I'm so grateful for the opportunity to be at these UCI points races and chase my Olympic qualification dream. It's just me and my little dream, trying to make our way through pelotons of six-person national teams. My inner joke is if there is one athlete I can relate to

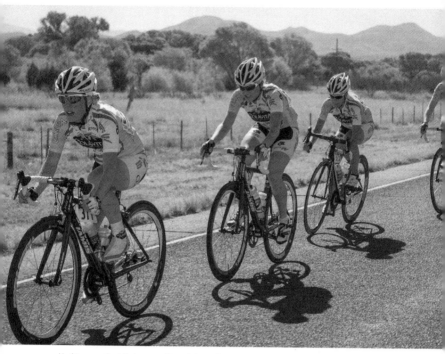

Nothing worthwhile is ever achieved alone. Sometimes it comes in triplicate. Or even quintuplicate. (Jonathan Devich/epicimages.us)

most, it would be U.S. soccer team goalkeeper Hope Solo.

Or in my case *Hope, Solo.*

You can imagine my surprise, then, when I received an email from a fellow pro cyclist I had never met before, offering to help me:

Hi Kathryn,

My name is Nicky Wangsgard. I'm a professor at Southern Utah University and professional cyclist. I race for Primal/ MapMyRide. I'm their sprinter. I'm also 39 and want to retire in one year. Need a teammate? Thought maybe I could help you

*qualify for an Olympic spot for St. Kitts and Nevis. Would love
to race with a purpose before I retire ...*

I knew Nicky by reputation—her self-description as a
"sprinter" was rather humble. During her 10-year career
in the sport, she has topped several podiums on the prestigious National Race Calendar circuit and collected a
wardrobe of coveted Most Aggressive jerseys. This was
one tough competitor—a tough competitor who, out of the
blue, wrote an email to a total stranger, offering to help her
reach the Olympics.

Hope, Duo!

It's one thing to want to help someone; it's a whole other
level of selflessness when a stranger says she's willing to
pay her own way, battle strange foreign circumstances, and
sacrifice her own ability to win all in the name of someone
else's dream. What a remarkable sport this was, sending
help my way at the eleventh hour of an Olympic dream. I
know now that angels exist, and they come dressed in lycra
and chamois.

Nicky and I checked the UCI race calendar. She would
be able to come with me to the four UCI races in Venezuela
in May 2012. *Perfect*, I thought. *Those are race courses I am
already familiar with, and I'll have a teammate to help me.* I was
all set. But I should know by now that whenever I think, *I'm
all set*, the opposite is usually true. Sure enough, another
glitch surfaced.

In the past, I've raced in Venezuela as a solo rider. This
year, I got an email explaining that if I wanted to come
to their UCI races, I'd need a minimum of four women to
comprise a team. Where was I going to find two more
women who were willing to spend thousands on a plane
ticket to a country with difficult logistics for racing,

eating, and sleeping, all for the glory of my own Olympic advancement?

Enter Hopes Trio and Quartet.

I learned one valuable lesson as a solo rider for one of cycling's underfunded nations: I am hardly alone. There are a lot of small nations with aspiring cyclists, yet they face the same struggles I do in attempting Olympic qualification. They have no teammates, no budget, and often no way of getting into races that require teams of four or more. So I contacted two of my fellow Olympic hopefuls in the same predicament as me: Claire Fraser from Guyana and Tamiko Butler from Antigua. I told the ladies we could help each other—if they came to Venezuela, they could race on my team and we'd total four women so they could chase their Olympic dreams, too.

Such composite teams offer a strange duality, as one's "teammates" are also one's competition. Far better, however, to be there as competitors than not at all. Maybe Tamiko or Claire would beat me and take the points I'm vying for. But unless we come to Venezuela together, we can't reach the start line at all. If there is one thing more important than my own Olympic dream, it is this: creating opportunity for change. Right now, the UCI caters to traditionally strong, deep-talent nations with centuries of cycling history, tradition, and pro teams, and they don't do much to help small countries with individual riders succeed or grow. But I can. Welcome to the Hope Show, Tamiko and Claire. May our voice be heard through our presence in Venezuela, whether we make it to the Games or not.

I was lucky to have a team of four, but I didn't expect a Hope Quintet. When Nicky's friend, Rachel Cieslewicz, came aboard as our fifth rider, I knew she represented the most important piece of the puzzle. In my intimate relationship with Murphy's Law, I know cycling well enough to predict that, with a team of four, it's far too likely someone will get sick or injured or have their bike lost in transit. Having Rachel swoop down in her angel chamois was the perfect antidote to potential problems.

As soon as I typed the words "potential problems," Mr. Murphy and his Law showed up in my inbox. Nicky was suddenly unable to go to Venezuela due to a family matter. With sheer selflessness and generosity, Nicky canceled her airline ticket and purchased one for her friend and fellow cyclist, Julie Cutts, to take her place so I would not be left stranded with too few teammates. The Quintet would remain intact, and I am silently reminded that goals of Olympic proportion are never accomplished alone.

Speaking of angels and chamois, we were in need of a team kit for Venezuela. While I race for Team Colavita domestically, my attempt to get to the Olympics falls under my own jurisdiction. Luckily, I race for one of the nicest organizations on the planet. John Profaci donated a few extra jerseys and bib shorts so the Hope Quintet will look the part of an official team. I've practically lost count of which Hope we're on, but I can think of no better words than *Hope, Fully* for the amount of help and true belief that has come my way. Then again, I'm pretty sure hope has been here all along.

THE ADVENTURES OF POCKETBABY
May 2012

IT'S A WARM SPRING MORNING in Tucson as I round the bend of our subdivision and head out on my training ride with my two-year-old daughter stuffed in my jersey pocket. She is eight inches tall. The birth took twenty-five minutes, the pregnancy not much longer. My little girl favors the right-side pocket so she can listen to the click and whir of the bicycle gears, and quite frankly, I prefer her to be on the inside of the bike lane anyway. It's safer. So there she stays, tucked in snug with her tiny head bobbing above the gentle cinch of the elastic pocket, and her tiny helmet visor shielding her from the morning sun, and gleeful exclamations of animals or pedestrians who catch her curious eyes. There is a plastic baggie of Cheerios for her and an energy bar for me. *Faster*, she cries. I hear my genes in her command.

After the ride, I go about the rest of my life with Pocketbaby in a similar manner, carrying her with me in my purse on all excursions outside the home. I treasure these years. After all, she'll bloom into a normal-size child in September of her sixth year, right in time for kindergarten. Till then, all the obstacles of early child rearing and simultaneously having my own life fit nicely in the palm of my hand. Or handbag.

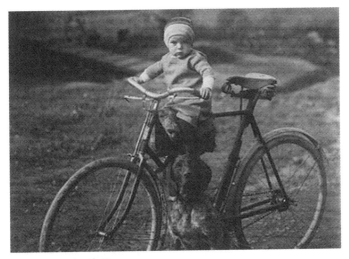

I'm ready for children. Really tiny ones.

○ ○ ○

This is the recurring dream I've had half a dozen times since my early thirties. We — this eight-inch child and I — are mostly on a bike, but the adventures of Pocketbaby vary to include other activities I enjoy. Sometimes we run or hike. Sometimes we meet with my publisher. Pocketbaby has excellent insight for a toddler.

"Mom," she pontificates from the purse, standing on my wallet so she can tug on my elbow. "I don't think it's wise to tell anyone about this dream."

"Ok, PB, you're mommy's little secret," I intone, my voice rising in the manner in which I speak to other people's strange-yet-lovely-looking pets. I give her a Cheerio. She wears it as a bracelet. We truly enjoy each other's company. I believe we'll be good friends upon adulthood.

And then I wake up from this particular installment of the Pocketbaby series, somewhere in the depths of rural Venezuela, cramped into a small hotel room with four other women and five bicycles. No babies of any size are present. It is Mother's Day. Two days ago, I celebrated my 37th birthday, furthering a certain disconnect between my brain and body. The latter believes I'm 25, and the former wants to agree but is bound by the truth, thus resulting in the lengthening pause when someone asks how old I am. My answer lilts with a tone of indecision. I'm…37?

The conception of Pocketbaby doesn't surprise me. I've always been an incredibly vivid dreamer. I've completed an octuple axel, securing my title as the world's most powerful figure skater. Taken down a fire-breathing dragon tormenting a small village with an upper cut I learned in a Gold's Gym kickboxing class. Recently, I auditioned for a modern ballet ensemble choreographed by The Rock. Damn straight I got the part. So it wasn't a shock when Pocketbaby showed up a few years ago.

It is impossible to mention Pocketbaby without divulging a different recurring dream I had when I was a child. In this dream series I had a younger brother named Philip. We played together, making mudpies and climbing trees, and he had to listen to me and do what I said because I was the big sister. In my real life family, my brother is seven year my senior. As children, my tangible brother and I didn't interact much, given the age and gender difference. I suppose I felt lonely, and thus my subconscious gave me Philip to play with in my dreams. They were nice, these dreams. Little Phil had a charming bowl haircut and was thrilled to be my playmate. He was clearly the psychological precursor to his future niece, Pocketbaby.

Also not surprising is that Pocketbaby's manifestation is a direct representation of my current indecision on whether to have my own biological, non-miniature children. I simply haven't gotten the call of motherhood, and I'm not sure if I'm supposed to be the one dialing or receiving. Enter into the mix these ingredients: a strained adult relationship with my own mother, an acute knowledge of just how much work is involved in childrearing, an odd yet palatable fear that unlike Pocketbaby, a real baby won't like me, and a husband that doesn't mind at all if we just stay us. So there we are. I'm not sure what to do with all that. Except to wait. And listen.

I have always loved children. Other people's. In high school, my less-than-stellar popularity led to a highly profitable weekend babysitting career. I really enjoyed spending time with kids, and for the most part I believe they liked me back. I didn't just "sit" for them. We ran and jumped and hid and played and engaged one another while dinner was made and bedtime stories were read. By the time my five-hour shift was over and I handed the kids back to their parents, I was thoroughly exhausted. At the age of 17, I fully understood how much work went into being a full-time parent, especially a very good one. My subconscious took note as well. *Might be a few years till we're ready to do that for free, it whispered.*

Twenty years later, my desire to have my own children (other than Pocketbaby) still has yet to surface. Should the baby urge surge for either George or myself, we'll revisit the topic. Yet for a woman nearing 40, biological reality creeps in now and then, complete with society's annoyingly prevalent list of Shoulds, Coulds, and Woulds. It would be safer to have a kid sooner than later. Should do it now, all my peers are on their second and third offspring. Motherhood could be the best decision I ever make. Yet stronger still remains this one Should in particular: If my gut tells me not to do something right now, shouldn't I obey my innermost truth mechanism?

Being Mother's Day, I'm not surprised Pocketbaby chose to recur near this particular calendar mark. In addition to thinking about kids, I also think about my moms. I have two. One is of the flesh (to whom I send a card), the other is Title IX (no card, but still grateful). Here, in the year Title IX turns 40, I can attest I'm a daughter of this movement. I took a road less traveled through the maze of women's sports, all because I had the opportunity and desire to do so. What started with a kickball homerun during a third-grade recess match has morphed into a pro cycling career in my late thirties. I'm not only in love with sport but the activism and betterment for it. Many sports, like women's cycling, still need some assistance in bushwhacking better trails of equality. Perhaps it is my calling to mother a movement rather than a child. Though someday, if I do have a daughter, I look forward to her blank stares of boredom as I jabber on about the poor pay scales, fewer race opportunities, and fight for media attention we had in women's cycling. Hope envision her rolling her eyes and saying, "Whatever, Mom, it's not like that now. Let's go, I'll be late for football practice."

On this particular Mother's Day in the heart of Venezuela, thoughts of what I should, would, or could be doing in regard to motherhood take a backseat to what actually is: I'm an athlete with a dream on a mission. What I am doing here in the depths of South America, racing for Olympic qualification points, is for me. There are no guarantees I'll make it. There are no guarantees I won't. Some people have the notion that slim-chance dreams and/or not having children is selfish and unrealistic. Yet lately I've come to believe that what I am doing is not only best for me but also the best thing I can do for my metaphorical maybe-child or for any kid that dares to dream big. I'm living my life, pursuing my goals and going after what I want without the promise of anything coming to fruition or going as planned. I am trying. Doing. Hoping. In my private universe of logic, trying is not only the greatest achievement and the most powerful action one can do with their lives, but also the lifelong antidote to the ailment of the What-Ifs.

These are the lessons I'd like to instill in my future children, whether they arrive into this world through my body, fertility clinics, adoption, foster care, or perhaps not at all and it ends up being other people's children I affect. So I can only hope Pocketbaby understands why mommy (or crazy Auntie Kathryn) is going to go race her bike today.

While I question just about everything on the topic of children, I do know is the one truth I've come to treasure through my off-the-beaten-path odyssey of adulthood: The gut knows all. Let go, and let Gut. My job is to listen to that strange internal thud of what feels right or wrong. I have to believe and trust that if my gut wants a child to occupy its lower quarters, then it will tell me so. Too many years have been spent on my proclivity, desire and rather exhausting need to figure out how the heart and brain and gut are connected. I've recently decided to retire from this role of emotional detective, and instead adopt the role of being a client in my own Life Decision firm. I'll let my gut call the shots and tell me when or if we're ever ready for motherhood. Or ready for anything, really. Choosing to listen to the gut however, doesn't make the Pocketbaby dreams go away or keep the tangled thoughts of parenting from forming. These, I'm guessing, are part of the gut's deliberation process. So for now, I look forward to my next nocturnal adventure with Pocketbaby. We'll see what comes next. Maybe she'll hit a growth spurt. Maybe I will. In the meantime, we'll hop on the bike and do our thing, with the sun on our faces, the wind in our hair, and the calm in our gut telling us this is exactly how it's supposed to be right now.

I shift my focus to my upcoming race in Venezuela where my teammates and I begin cleaning the grime from yesterday's race off our bikes, getting ready for today's event. In some parts of the world, bicycles are synonymous with childhood. In this particular hotel room, bicycles are synonymous with the betterment of five female adult-hoods, ranging in age from 21 to 44. We're all racing our bikes for different reasons; beginning a pro career, ending a pro career, pursuing Olympic qualification points, helping others get their goals. We're all racing our bikes for the same reason; something from the past or dreams of the future has drawn us to the life of physical effort and athleticism, and it has told us to keep going. Two of us are moms. Three of us are childless. We're all happy. At this very moment in time, we're all doing exactly what our gut tells us we're supposed to be doing—reveling in the present.

INEXPERIENCE IS NOT THE SAME AS WEAKNESS
May 2012

FOUR YOUNG WOMEN from the Panamanian national team are packing up their bicycles, disassembling the frames, and loading them into bulky plastic cases required for airplane transport. I'm confused, though. We've only raced two of the four UCI races here in Venezuela. We still have two to go. I ask why they are leaving early. Don't they want to shoot for those elusive Olympic qualification points?

They do, but there's problem. The race director is sending them home. Of the six international teams represented in Venezuela, only the Panamanian team was required to stay at a different hotel in a different city, a hotel more than an hour away from the rest of the teams. The Venezuelan federation, which pays for all international teams' hotel rooms during the events, wanted to lessen their expenses and requested the Panamanian team move to a cheaper hotel. But the Panamanian women did not feel safe in a strange city so far from the other riders, and the roads and riding routes were unfamiliar.

"Why does our team have to go?" they asked. The answer: politics. Panama placed last as a team in our first two races. A minimum of five international teams are

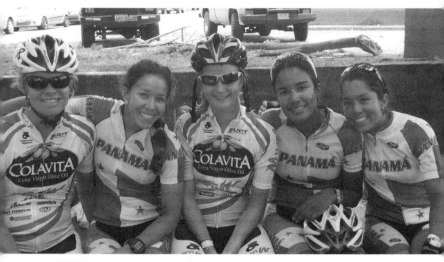

The Panamanian development team gives a great lesson in the state of women's cycling; we're all vying for equality.

required for UCI points races, and Panama brought that number to six. In finishing last, the Panamanians had become superfluous. When they tried to argue that they belonged in the same hotel as the rest of the competitors, or at least in a location where they felt safe, the Venezuelan federation refused and sent the Panamanians home.

My teammate, Julie, and I watched them pack. It didn't feel right. I was in their shoes four years ago as an inexperienced rider just trying to keep up with the big dogs and was often last in the races. I've been broomwagoned in Europe, dropped in the United States, and crashed out in corners of the Caribbean and Central America, but no one ever told me to go home or moved me to unsafe locations.

Julie and I told the Panamanian women they could have our hotel room and we'd purchase separate accommodations. The ladies thanked us, but their pride had been wounded and their plane reservations already changed.

"We came for the experience of racing, but because we are weak, we are no longer wanted here," said Lianna, a young Panamanian rider. "It's time to leave."

Feeling powerless against the politics of the sport, all I could do was correct them on one major point.

"Inexperience is not the same as weakness," I offered, urging the young women to keep racing and to use their disappointment as fuel for training. Don't quit over controversy, I begged them. Keep riding. Someday your country will have an Olympic cyclist. The more I spoke, the more I realized just how personal this issue had become. As I've raced internationally for St. Kitts and Nevis during the past four years, I've competed in a lot of remote places and seen a lot of eye-opening behaviors. I've witnessed course-cutting cheaters, sketchy race directors, touchy-feely creepy coaches, commissaries with a penchant for posting rather creative race results, and routes laden with precarious potholes and uncovered sewer openings.

The sport has its obstacles, but the one obstacle we must overcome is speaking out on issues of fairness and growth for women's cycling. It is not okay to invite a young national team to a UCI event and then send them home because they are "last." It is not okay to cater only to today's winners and mistake the next generation's temporary inexperience as weakness. It is not okay to discourage women in sport. I am not okay with what happened to the Panamanians. Every cyclist—every *athlete* in every *sport*—starts out as Panama. We must stick up for the beginners; they are our future.

Now, more than ever, we must show the inconsistencies

and inequalities in women's sports and rally against them. Of course, politics are everywhere in sport and always will be, but that doesn't mean we should accept such discourse. Phrases like "Life's not always fair" are often tossed around with dismissive nonchalance, but fairness and life are not the correct pairing. Life can occasionally be crappy or less than lucky, but fairness is not a trait of chance or even biology—it is a conscious choice and characteristic of people. *People* decided Panama couldn't race anymore. *People* took away their Olympic qualification dreams. *People* sent them home. Hopefully, *people* can set this right. There will be some who attempt to rescind the progress of women's sports, but I believe there will be more who band together and help it grow. It will be people, ultimately, who build the road of equality and decide where it will lead.

THAT'S BIKE RACING
April 2012

IN CYCLING, THERE IS THE PHRASE we use to shrug off the complexities and challenges of our sport. Got a flat tire in a really important race? Break your collarbone after overlapping wheels with a competitor? Lose your water bottles after running over a nasty pothole? *That's bike racing.*

I rather dislike this phrase. The annoying accuracy and honesty of it robs me of the chance to wallow in misery when something goes wrong. Granted, I've never been one to wallow, but I find it far more effective for my mental health to verbally release the momentary frustration of a tough race situation. When we stub our toe on a chair leg, it's normal to let loose an expletive or two. I've never heard anyone cry out, "Well, that's furniture."

And so, under the banner of all that is good and bad in bike racing, here's how my week at the 2012 UCI Energiewacht Tour in Holland went—starting with how I got there but my bike did not.

Upon returning from a stage race in El Salvador, I got a last-minute invitation to join the Dutch team called Water, Land & Dijken for the prestigious UCI event in Northern Holland, where I would have six stages and five days to chase those elusive Olympic qualification points. Because I had a stopover in St. Kitts and Nevis on the way back from

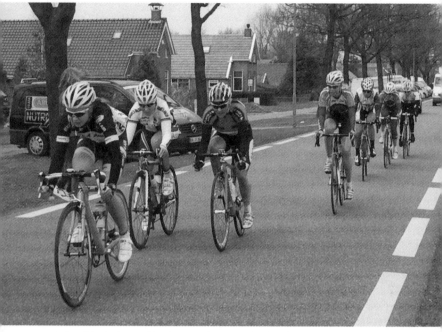

A shot of the third stage of the Energiewacht Tour in Holland. As for why I'm snapping the picture instead of being in the race, well. . .that's bike racing.

El Salvador (including a lot of connecting flights, baggage fees, and delayed luggage hazards), it made more sense to ship my bike home from El Salvador via FedEx so it would be there in time for me to dash off to Holland. This was all well and good until the call came from my husband, George: "Honey, FedEx can't find your bike. Or your wheel box. They have no record of either."

As much as I would have loved to say, "Well, that's FedEx" and let the whole thing go, that sentiment was not an option. Not with an Olympic dream hanging in the balance. Instead, we delegated tasks. George dealt with FedEx and the nagging fact that $10,000 worth of sports equipment had vanished. I dealt with how I was going to race without a bicycle.

There were two main options: a) Don't go to Holland; or b) Don't be an idiot; my Olympic dream is at stake, so borrow a bike and go to Holland.

Trying to find a bike to borrow in 48 hours isn't easy. For one, most people don't have high-end spare bikes lying around that they eagerly lend out to others. Second, I also needed a bike travel case, which was also lost. So I did what I usually do in times of emergency and need: I logged on to Facebook and Twitter. Remarkably, within three hours, two possible solutions came through. My friend, Chris Jeffrey, a pro triathlete who was out for a few weeks with a broken collarbone, had a road bike and a travel case for me. Then, a seemingly even better offer came through! A bike store in Holland had a top-of-the-line bike they'd lend me for the race.

"You won't have to fly with your bike, just come on over!" they said, asking for my frame size and specific measurements. I sent them over. We were all set.

Upon arriving in Holland, where the incredibly lovely Kessler family took me in and shuttled me to the race (2.5-hour drive from the airport), I had about 24 hours until the first stage, a time trial. Luckily, my time trial bike was not lost to the void of international shipping. I used Chris' bike case to bring my TT bike to Holland, and it served me well. On the cold, gray, windy day in Appingedam, I felt amazingly strong in a very specific manner I refer to as the Keavy Effect.

My friend, Keavy McMinn, let me use her airline miles to upgrade to business class on the way to Holland. I had one of those nifty seat-turns-into-bed arrangements, not usually found in my back-of-the-plane, middle-seat travel budget to which I'm accustomed. This remarkable chair-bed luxury was a major benefit, as dealing with a last-minute flight, jet lag, and a race within 24 hours can be physically debilitating for any racer. Being able to lie down for most of the journey was a key factor to a very good race result.

I placed 57th out of 150 women in the time trial. While most people would wince that I used "57th" and "very good" in the same breath, bike racing isn't like most sports. While there are rarely 57 marathoners, triathletes, or race-walkers who cross the finish line in the course of one minute, cycling is different. In this race, less than 90 seconds separated the competitors from the top 10 to the top 60. For me, it was further proof that I am getting better and faster. *Man, this Olympic dream really is such a great fairy tale in the making!* I couldn't wait for the road race. That's where the fairy tale turned from Disney to Grimm.

I knew something was a little off when I picked up the borrowed road bike I'd be racing for the remainder of the stages. Beautiful as the snazzy carbon-fiber steed was, the handlebars looked a bit big. So did the bike length.Flicking out my nerdy travel tape measure, my suspicions were confirmed. "Not quite" in cycling measurements is not a good thing. It's like giving a runner the wrong size shoes at the start of a marathon. Yet under the circumstances, it didn't bother me. I was *there*. I would *race*. That's all that mattered. So what if I needed to be about a foot taller for this particular bike? There were 16 hours until the first road race. I could grow. I've always had an excellent ability to use positive(ly unrealistic) rationalization when necessary. Besides, it wasn't like the bike was going to fall apart or anything.

The temperature in Papenburg, Holland, at the start of the road race was 35 degrees, and the women in the peloton shook with cold. The howling wind and fierce competition should have been my main competitors. Instead, my nemesis became a 65-cent seat-post bolt that quietly began to cry mutiny, slowly unwinding its dedication to my dream. After a section of rough cobblestones, the seat post slipped five centimeters. My knees bowed out, and so did all my power. My road bike had become as powerful as a tricycle. I began to slide back from the middle of the peloton...back, back, back...away from the pack, then alone on the roads, back further still until I saw an old friend. Hello, broom wagon, how nice to see you again.

The broom wagon is the car that sweeps away the dropped riders, the ones who have no chance of winning, asking for our race numbers and, in doing so, officially severing our umbilical cord to the peloton. The mechanical difficulties of my seat post left me time cut, which meant I was no longer allowed to complete the upcoming stages of the race. I had been in Holland for 36 hours, and there would be no more hopes for Olympic qualification points. The 10-hour flight, the 20-minute time trial, the jet lag, the borrowed bike, the poor results, and the disappointment throbbed deep within my mind and searched for a way out, but I was surrounded by strangers and teammates and had to play the maturity card.

"That's bike racing," I offered, staving off tears.

But my heart had stubbed its toe and gave a silent temper tantrum only I could hear:

Sometimes I really hate this sport. It really sucks. I hate FedEx. I hate it when stuff doesn't turn out the way I want. I worked really hard. I hate that a half-inch piece of metal has any say in my dreams. I hate being polite. Polite sucks. I don't want to sit down and relax; I want to throw this stinkin' broken bike across the flippin' race course. I hate the word "flippin'." Only polite people say that. I hate that I had to say thank you to the guy who lent me the bike when I really wanted to curse him out for it falling apart because I am angry and blame helps right now and I don't wanna be mature. I'm tired and I'm hungry and sore and the peanut butter in Holland tastes like crap and I'm still mad at that girl in eighth grade who stole my summer-camp boyfriend and I really miss my childhood dog and...

Whoa, okay. Maybe "That's bike racing" isn't such a bad phrase after all. I had not considered its potential as a protective dam for emotional floods. Mostly, though, I dislike the phrase because it's only applied to the negative things we encounter in racing. Yes, indeed, bad stuff happens in bike racing like it does in any aspect of life in general. Still, I'd rather the phrase be used for helping us remember the benefits of our sport, especially when times get tough.

Flying business class to Europe for a chance to chase my dreams. Having friends lend me their equipment, money, time, and energy because they believe in me. A family of strangers taking me into their home. A foreign team letting me race for them. A time trial with promise and potential. The bone-chilling cold weather on race day reminding me I'm alive. The seat-post screw reminding me that effort and circumstance might not always align, but showing up to try still counts for something. Doing something—anything—with our life is the gift of sport, regardless of the result. Still having a shot at your goals, picking yourself up, trying again (and again and again), and getting back on the bike...

Now *that's* bike racing.

ROCK. AND ROLL.
November 2011

ONE OF MY GREATEST NON-CYCLING passions is film. Watching movies, studying them, writing screenplays, accepting imaginary Oscars…oh, how I love film. When my cycling off-season rolls around, I actually have the time to catch up on my beloved indie flicks and off-the-beaten-path documentaries. Every October and November, I glue myself to the couch, heave my achin' legs onto some pillows, and run up the Apple TV bill.

The other day I watched *Anvil! The Story of Anvil*, Sacha Gervasi's 2008 documentary about the 1980s Canadian heavy metal band called, well, Anvil. The band was a leader in the music industry, paving the way for metal greats like Metallica, Guns N' Roses, and Anthrax.

Now, I am not a heavy metal fan. Nor do I gravitate toward drug-inclined, frizzy-haired men in their fifties. Not to mention my personal recollections of the '80s are less glam rock and more *Fraggle Rock*. *Anvil!*, it seemed, would necessitate some Advil. But I watched it anyway. And absolutely melted.

I love this movie.

Only in explaining the plot to my husband did I come to understand how Anvil had struck such a chord with me, a female athlete in her mid-thirties who listens to Bob Dylan.

119

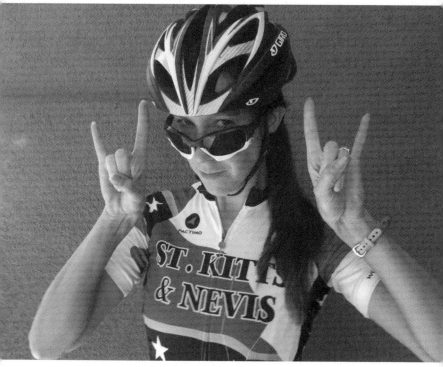

Inspired by washed up old metalheads? Absolutely! (George Varhola)

"See, George, it's about this heavy metal band that was so passionate about its craft, but they ran into all these logistical nightmares in terms of management, and while their contemporaries were making it big, they faltered in securing bookings and all this basic tactical stuff. But even now, all these years past their prime, they're still trying to make it happen. They're so passionate about their music, and they work so hard, and they're giving it everything they have, and they're still not giving up about making it to the 'big stage...'"

That's when it hit me. My God. I *am* Anvil. On wheels.

Anvil's still trying to make it to the big stage; I'm on my second attempt at Olympic qualification. Anvil is old for a band; I am old-ish for an Olympic hopeful. Anvil has trouble getting booked; I have to constantly harass UCI race directors to let me into qualifying events. They've slept in European train stations; I've slept in South American airports. Lead singer Steve "Lips" Kudlow's day job is driving a truck that delivers middle school lunch food. To fund my athletic dreams, I worked three years as a middle school substitute teacher and likely ate that very food. What are the chances? *I truly understand you, Anvil, you beautiful, persistent weirdos.*

All of a sudden, it was no longer strange that my kindred brothers were four old heavy metal rockers who wear Borat-approved leather clothing and play slide guitars with sexual devices. In fact, at the end of the movie, Anvil shot to the top five on my Lottery List. You know, the list of people and things you'd like to help if you won the lottery? *The homeless. The hungry. The sick. Global media equality for women's sports. Anvil.*

Here, in this little indie documentary, I found a surprising affirmation of my life journey. The film isn't about heavy metal. It isn't about four dudes in a band or a hard-rock lifestyle. It's about having a dream and sticking to it. It's about believing in oneself. It's about entertaining goals of greatness while coping with reality. It's about merging inner drive with driving a catering truck to make it all happen. It's about fighting the Triple Ds: doubters, don't-ers, and inner demons. It's about having heart, no matter how many times it may get ripped out of your chest. It's about coming in last and having the courage to find your way to the next starting line. It's about *knowing* you have what it takes to win even if no one else thinks you do…and that you'll get there, eventually.

As far as I'm concerned, the members of Anvil are honorary athletes. At least metaphorically. And not just athletes—they symbolize anyone who has ever reached for the stars in any universe of talent. From Sundance to Sydney to Los Angeles, film festival audiences were as touched as I was, repeatedly honoring *Anvil!* with the prestigious Audience Choice award.

In about three months, my 2012 Olympic qualification attempt will be in full swing. I'll be just like Anvil, going on tour with my one-woman band of dreams. El Salvador, Belgium, Venezuela, I'll perform in places with few spectators, putting on a show for which there are no tickets, no stadium seating, no audience. Just a girl on a bike. When the tough days come, the pain sets in, and the doubts arise, I—an English major with a 15-year journalism career—won't seek inspiration from Emerson, Churchill, or Molière. Instead, I'll be carrying the words of a 50-year-old metal head named Lips in my heart:

"Always believe that no matter how hard it gets, there's always a way."

Thanks, Anvil. From one dream chaser to another: You keep rocking, I'll keep rolling.

ON TAKING
May 2011

MY FRIEND, DIANE, once suggested that I'm brave for following my Olympic dreams. "It takes guts to go all around the world and go for something so big with no guarantee you'll get it," she reasoned, citing my globetrotting quest to win Olympic qualification points.

I laughed and dismissed such "braveness" as nothing more than an inner drive and passion to see how far I can go in this sport (and this life). *I'm not brave*, I thought to myself. *Just determined. And a wee bit stubborn.* But that was before my recent trip to Venezuela. I think I might be brave now.

Olympic qualification points can only be gained at certain elite/pro-level races hosted by the Union Cycliste Internationale, or UCI. To get into these races, a cyclist either needs a sanctioned UCI team or an invitation. So if I'm lucky enough to find a UCI team to let me guest ride, or garner a coveted invitation, I go wherever that race may be: Belgium, Holland, Colombia. After eight weeks competing in foreign countries this past spring, I gained incredible strength, power, and speed, but alas, no points.

Only the top eight finishing racers get points, and sometimes as many as 200 women show up to the races. Sometimes the participation number is less, but the racers are no less vicious. In a pre-Olympic year, everyone wants

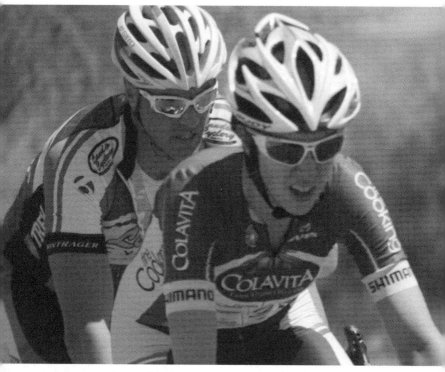

Sometimes you have to ask for what you want in life. Sometimes you have to take it.
(Alyosha Boldt)

points, and there are no easy races. My best finish was 12th at the Pan Am Championships in Medellin, Colombia, last week. Qualification points went to the top eight.

Close, but there are no points for closeness. Nor is there aspirin specific to this type of brain pain.

When I got the approval to race in Venezuela last weekend, I was thrilled albeit a little petrified. I'd have to go alone and rely on the Venezuelan Cycling Federation to pick me up, help me find housing, and generally point me in the direction of the start lines for its two road race events. In other sports, being a pro athlete is seen as luxurious. Women's cycling, however, has a long way to go.

Venezuelans are kind, warm, wonderful people…who speak very, very quickly. No one in the Venezuelan federation spoke English, but I had just enough high school Spanish left in my memory to communicate/pantomime, as long as the conversation stayed in the present tense and I asked them to speak *muy despacio*. I had been to Venezuela in 2008 for some races. Perhaps they'd remember me, the girl representing "St. Kittens and Novice."

The journey to Venezuela started with two flights from Colombia and then a seven-hour car trip to a tiny rural town south of Caracas. The man driving me was a complete stranger sent to fetch me from the Venezuelan Cycling Federation, and the roads were harrowing, twisty, and without lighting. Many South American highways— Venezuela notwithstanding—are rather frightening, as lane lines and stop signs appear to be nothing more than decorative. Taillights are optional, and overtaking trucks by crossing the double yellow line is a common practice. Adding to this conundrum, the man driving me was texting, drowsy, and constantly misplacing his glasses. He also had early-onset Parkinson's.

Diane's words echoed in my head. But the bravery notion didn't really kick in until we got to the village of Aricagua and I was dropped off at a motel at 11:30 PM. There were inebriated people stumbling in the hallway, my door lock didn't work, the toilet needed to be manually filled with water before use, a bird living in the air conditioner sent twigs cascading onto my pillow, and large patches of mold and paint chips blotched the ceiling.

"I think my hotel is nicer than yours," the driver said, as he left me in the lobby and drove to the four-star hotel where the race directors were staying. In an effort to save money, many federations are fond of booking athletes in separate (read: lesser) accommodations. "Lock the door," he whispered.

As I lay in my decrepit bed, it dawned on me it had been hours since I'd eaten—and it would be a total of 17 hours of foodlessness before someone came to get me the next day. The paint chips began to look tasty. I refrained.

In my race the next day, I finished 11th—just three spots away from gaining some qualification points. Tired, depleted, and far from home, I began to question myself. Was the dream really worth it? I'd been on this quest for nearly four years now. All the difficult travel, all the time away from my husband, all the heartbreak of finishing close-but-no-cigar? Points seemed impossible. The doubt that began to creep into my head couldn't be quieted. Sometimes believing in yourself is exhausting. Dogged by fatigue, my doubt and confidence battled it out:

I'm 36, enough already. You're racing stronger than ever.

This kind of racing is hard to do alone. It's harder to look back and wonder, "What if?"

I used to go into every race thinking I had a chance, but now I don't know anymore. Then turn your brain off and listen to your body. It knows what to do.

Sometimes I'm afraid of my own dream.

You don't have to get over your fear in order to do something. It's okay to bring the fear with you. Just cut out its tongue first.

I'm hungry. There's a dude selling empanadas on the street. Be brave.

The next day, on the start line of my final Venezuelan race, I decided it was time to stop believing and to start doing. I wasn't tired or sad or philosophical or optimistic.

I was pissed.

Doubt was getting on my nerves, and I had to do something about it. Wanting points wasn't enough. No one was going to hand them to me. No one else cared how much I traveled, how much I trained, how much I truly wanted to reach my goals. Enough with all this points wanting. It was time for points taking.

For the next two hours, I went after what I wanted with more confidence than any race I've had in the past. I attacked up hills, led on the descents, pushed the pace on the flats. My finishing sprint is not my strongest discipline, so when the inevitable came, I dug deep into the SoulBowels—that inner place where a cyclist's physical effort rattles their intestines and inner being—and crossed the line in sixth place. My highest UCI finish.

After years of trying, I finally had the points I so desperately wanted. Eight of them! Not enough to get "St. Kills and Navis"—this year's creative translation—a berth to the Games yet, but I still have one more year of point collecting. This is a very good start. Or perhaps, it's actually a very good end—the end of doubt, the restart of confidence, and a continuation of bravery.

After all, my vision-impaired, textaholic Venezuelan driver and I still have a treacherous seven-hour drive back to the Caracas airport. Even that fear can't take away the joy of knowing I'm one step closer to London.

ON NUTS, NEARLIES, AND KICKING BACK

January 2012

AS A WRITER, I pride myself in choosing wise, insightful words when putting my life into paragraph form. But then, there's my inner athlete; she prefers the more direct approach. So I'm letting her write this piece about our recent encounter with disappointment, struggle, and heartache as we attempt to qualify for the 2012 London Olympics: I just got kicked in the nuts.

At least that's how it feels. Female athletes aren't supposed to talk that way. But for an athlete, male or female, sometimes that's exactly how disappointment feels when it comes on the heels of unfairness—like a kick to the most vulnerable part of our being. Before we get to the kicking part, here's some background.

In June 2011, I won my third straight time trial and road race national championship for St. Kitts and Nevis, the country of which I am a dual-citizen and represent as a cyclist. The latest win at nationals was important in a pre-Olympic year, especially for a small nation like mine that has not yet earned an Olympic berth in cycling. As the winner, I received 10 Olympic qualification points in the road race and three for the time trial, as allotted by the

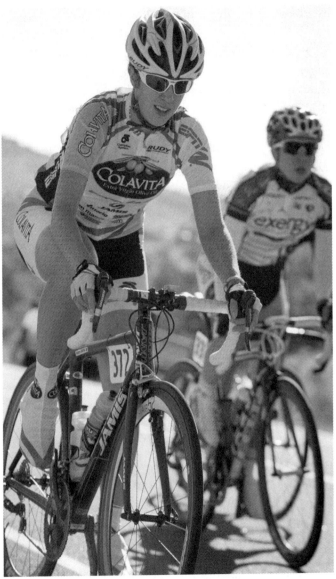

At some point, getting kicked down is part of every athletic journey. So is learning how to kick back.

International Cycling Union (UCI), the sport's governing body.

These qualification points are very hard to get. Racers all over the world value them like Golden Tickets. If I earn enough UCI points to rank within the top 100 by May 31, 2012, St. Kitts and Nevis receives a cycling berth for the Olympics. I have been chasing this dream for six years. Between my national championship points and the eight points I won during a UCI race in Venezuela, I had 21 UCI points. It was enough to rank me No. 125 in the world...a very doable position for reaching the top 100 by the end of May.

So a few weeks later, when I went to check the UCI standings to see what my competition was up to, I got a little confused when I didn't see my name where it had once been. Had I slipped down in the rankings? Oh well, it happens. Yet reading through the entire rankings of more than 400 women who had earned points, revealed that my name was nowhere. *Typo*, my inner writer thought, as I composed an email to the UCI to inquire, while a hollow ache of unease grew in my gut. *There's no typo, sweetheart*, my inner athlete intimated.

Brace yourself.

After weeks of badgering, the UCI eventually returned my emails. The governing body had taken away my points. Although the Venezuela race was listed as a UCI points race and the points had already been given out, the UCI ruled not enough international teams had participated and rescinded the eight points I won there. (Apparently, what the UCI giveth, the UCI taketh away.)

I winced at the reality. It's unbelievable how so much is out of our control when it comes to our very own dreams.

My disappointment was overwhelming, but I consoled myself with one reality: at least I still had my national championship points.

Then came the really big groin kick: the UCI would no longer count my 13 national championship points because the St. Kitts and Nevis federation sent in the results two days late for a deadline unbeknownst to it. Our federation is new, small, and humble, and still learning the intricacies of the UCI. It was unaware of any deadline and had not received an email or letter stating such a rule. To this, the UCI responded, "Well, you're not alone. There were plenty of other countries that didn't get points for the same reason."

Not exactly comforting. Not exactly right. A national champion potentially not qualifying for the Olympics because of an email mistake? That's not okay.

I argued. I fought. I got nowhere with the UCI. Then I did what anyone does when a dream is rendered nearly impossible. I cried. Dry heaved. Cried some more. Wallowed in the disappointment. And then I did what any athlete does when they hear the world "nearly." I used it to rebuild. Nearly impossible is not the same as impossible. It's time to start again. Not at No. 125 or even No. 400. I'll have to start from nothing and travel the world for the next two months, attempting to regain what I'd lost.

It's a daunting road, navigating this physical and emotional path through "kicks" and "nearly."

My husband, George, brings much-needed comfort. Slowly, he puts up emotional scaffolding around my Olympic dreams and reminds me there is still time. He reminds me I am riding and racing stronger than he's ever seen; a setback doesn't mean game over; lost points *can* be regained. It is up to me now to get past the pain and believe in myself again. This seems like a job for my inner athlete. I ask if she knows how, exactly, I'm supposed to get back on track.

You got kicked in the...

"Yeah, I know. Not helpful."

Let me finish. You got kicked in the heart. You got kicked in the head. You got kicked in the soul and in the spaces where disappointment hurts an athlete most. But you still have your legs. So kick back.

The switch flips. My sadness turns a corner and runs smack into self-reliance. No matter the mental obstacles, an athlete is still in control of her body, and that has to be enough. I *do* have my legs, and should the UCI ever rip them off, I've got plenty of duct tape. So, here and now, I'm kicking back.

On the bike today, I kicked out the last of the sadness. I kicked out the burdens outside my control. I kicked myself into a reestablished dream. I kicked out higher watt averages than I have all year. I knew nothing good would come from kicking the governing body of my sport. What's done is done. So instead, I kicked Doubt in the nuts. And I laughed while it cried.

So go ahead, UCI, take away my points. I'll get more. And while you're at it, take my disappointment, my heartache, and my frustration. I don't need those, either. Here are some other things you can take:

Take the high road when it comes to helping federations that are still growing in the sport of cycling.

Take caution when taking away what an athlete's earned.

Take care of your cyclists, fight for them and not against.

But above all, take note: Game on.

I'll see you in London.

GIVE ME SOMETHING TO BELIEVE IN
February 2012

MY OLYMPIC QUEST points debacle seemed to touch a nerve in the cycling community. A good nerve, apparently—one that brought much support and positive feedback from fellow cyclists and cycling fans as I attempt to regain my UCI ranking and shoot for Olympic qualification. It provided just the kind of mental edge I needed to regroup and move forward after a setback. A non-cycling buddy of mine asked if, in the wake of disappointment, getting back on the bike and rerouting the dream made long training days that much harder.

"All those hours on the bike, when you're out there for five hours by yourself, where does your mind go?" she asked. "When the odds are stacked against you, do the negative thoughts get in there while you're training? How do you kick them out?"

Valid questions. Every athlete in every sport has training days when their mind defeats them before their body even sets foot on the field, track, road, pool, or court. It's part of the athletic journey, and so is flipping the emotional switch and finding a way to derail any negative train of thought. Recently, I've found a great way to work around doubt and disappointment by doing something very simple: believing.

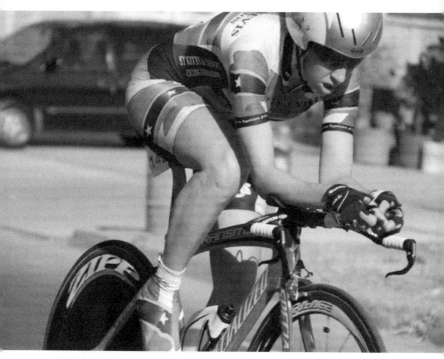

Believing in yourself can be downright exhausting. Sometimes it helps to believe in other things. Like Hostess cupcakes.

I don't mean believing in myself. Sure, an athlete has to believe in herself, but sometimes it's just too much to force-feed the mind another pep talk about how awesome you think you are, or how "you can do it" or how you're going to get up that hill. That's exhausting. On the days when feeling less than awesome, it is sometimes best to leave oneself alone and find something else to believe in. Luckily, there's a lot out there.

During my five-hour training ride the other day, I took some mental notes on some things I currently believe in or find inspiring. In random order, here's a starter list of what rolls through my head as I cycle through the desert landscapes:

- I believe Tucson might be the greatest place on the planet to train in the middle of February.
- Like the old children's cartoon where the hungry, delirious, shipwrecked man looks at his buddy and sees instead a giant, dancing turkey drumstick…I believe that every person ahead of me on our local group rides is not a person but an animated UCI point I must chase down.
- I believe the UCI can do better for its female athletes and developing nations, and we must continue to speak out on injustices and inequalities until we get what we deserve.
- I believe there will someday be women's road cycling world champions who hail from Africa, Asia, South America, and the Caribbean. It is a question of "when," not "if."
- I believe the Tour de France is missing an enormous financial, social, and moral opportunity by not allowing a women's pro race to coincide with the men's event dates and distances.
- I believe, at 36, I'm stronger than I ever was at 19. Or 35. Age and athleticism don't have to be enemies.
- I believe the journey of Olympic pro cyclist Evelyn Stevens stands for something greater than we realize. Stevens' well-known story of leaving a Wall Street career at 26 to become a pro bike racer—after she got on a bike recreationally—who won nearly every U.S. pro race that year and soon became a national champion isn't just a cool story. Her self-discovery proves an excellent point: opportunity is everything. (So is having the guts to embrace an unknown talent and turn it into something greater.) I believe there is an Evelyn Stevens in every nation, and we

can find her if we give women of developing nations a chance to ride and race.

• I believe my second-place finish behind Stevens at the Valley of the Sun time trial showed me this whole "believing" thing works.

• I believe it's time for a lifetime ban on the first offense for athletes who cheat with performance-enhancing drugs.

• I believe in stopping to fill up water bottles at a gas station mini-mart and leaving with the entire Hostess cupcake display.

• I believe a long ride on a bicycle can detox the soul. Unless you have a saddle sore—then your soul kind of hates you for a few weeks.

• I believe the fat old dude with the fluorescent vest, clip-on mirror, and $15,000 Colnago drafting off me while telling me I'm "pretty fast for a lady" should probably be thanked. People like him make it possible for bike companies to sponsor pro athletes and teams.

• I believe professional female cyclists need to champion each other by sharing race results, press releases, and one another's greatness. (Even though, deep inside, we want to rip each other's legs off and it isn't always easy to salute the winners when we lose.) If one female racer is in the headlines for the right reasons, our whole sport moves forward.

• I believe Title IX was a great start, but until women's sports share the same media attention, salaries, and social influence their male counterparts enjoy, we should not rest on Title IX's laurels but instead seek our journey into Title Next.

• I believe that even on the days when I don't believe in myself, someone else usually does. So I just believe in them.

• I believe no athlete will ever reach their true potential until they encounter hardship and learn how to come back from it.

• I believe I can get to London.

• I believe I just put my dirty jersey into the wash with a Hostess cupcake still in the pocket.

And that, I believe, is a good place to stop believing. But only for today.

DNF VS. DNS
June 2012

TWO WEEKS AGO, I raced my final stage of the Exergy Tour in Idaho and crossed the line in less than first place. I knew immediately I had not earned enough qualification points to make it to London, and my Olympic dream, more than six years in the making, was over.

I remember rain, sadness, fatigue, and disappointment, but I recall few other details about the day except for my father's phone call that night as I packed up my things in the Holiday Inn of Boise. I thought he was calling to give me one of his great pep talks about being proud of my efforts and how I'm always a winner even if I come in 197th place, the typical, wonderful, supportive-dad-stuff. I wasn't prepared for the news of his impending open-heart surgery, just days away.

"I didn't want to tell you until your final qualification race was over," he said. "I wanted you to focus on your dream."

Oh, Dad. Really?!

A major (yet gentle) scolding for withholding such life-and-death information ensued, making sure he understood no dream ever surpassed the importance of a loved one's health. I bought a red-eye plane ticket to New York.

It took a few hours to gather my thoughts, as my father's

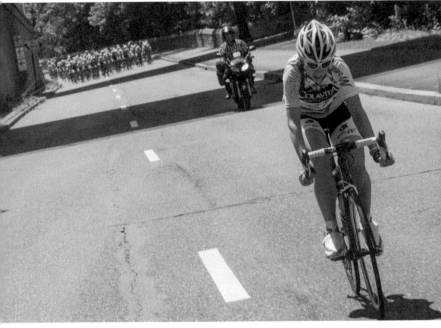

DNF: Did Not Finish. DNS: Did Not Start. The former always wins. (Jonathan Devich/ epicimages.us)

upcoming heart surgery and the finale of my Olympic dream ping-ponged my emotions. The state of my father's health dwarfed my disappointment on the bike, and I knew any frustration over the latter would release itself in its own time. And so, in the middle of a crowded Boise restaurant during our team dinner that evening, it did.

Somewhere between appetizers and entrées, time slowed down just enough for a reflection on the day, and the re-realization of my Olympic dream coming to an end. With public weeping in restaurants located near the bottom on my list of Fun Things in Life, I excused myself and let the disappointment run its course in private. But at the same time, I could see the Big Picture of what I had and had not achieved. Underneath the tears, everything really was okay. I've been through disappointment before; I'm familiar with the effects.

I have twice tried to cycle my way to the Olympics and did not succeed on either attempt. And yet, I refuse to use the word "fail." Not reaching a goal is one thing, but to attach failure to it would take away all I did achieve along the journey. From seeing the world to meeting incredible competitors to improving as an athlete, I have only gained, not lost. To "fail" at anything means one must first *try* something, so technically failure cannot exist without trying; and if there is effort, then perhaps there is no such thing as failure.

I believe trying—trying anything!—is what we are meant to do with our lives, and perhaps the only true failure is to never try. My father taught me this when he took up the sport of triathlon 10 years ago at age 66. He wasn't after a podium spot or an Olympic dream; he only wanted to partake in the greatest thrill of athleticism, which we so often overlook: trying.

Of course, that doesn't mean trying is easy; sometimes it's downright devastating. I compete in a sport that has a Broom Wagon—an actual car with brooms as decorations that sweeps losing cyclists off the course if they're not fast enough that day. It's rather humiliating. To commit to a life of pro cycling requires an athlete to sign a mental contract that states:

I am okay with being swept off European courses, dealing with hypercompetitive type-A women, having airlines lose/crack/ charge my bike, picking asphalt out of my thighs and getting my butt kicked on a regular basis, all for a 3-in-200 chance of stand-ing on a podium.

On many levels, cycling is a sport that practically ensures disappointment. And yet, those of us who love bike racing willingly sign that emotional contract time and time again because, at the core of it all, our soul somehow understands there is true beauty hidden in disappointment.

The gift of disappointment is it shows us our capac-ity to care, to want, to hope, and to be truly invested in life and go after our ambitions. It hurts when we don't reach our goal, but disappointment is an odd sort of vic-tory; it can be felt only by those who try. I put my heart and soul into trying. I am pretty certain that is what hearts and souls are for. There is no greater regret than looking back on life and wondering, "What if?" So, here I am at the end of a six-year adventure—and about 20 years of roads less taken—holding my head high, not as an Olympian, but as a proud Almostian. I do not regret one minute of my life-changing journey. London called, and I answered. We had a four-year conversation. I treasure every word, sentiment, and lesson learned from our *tête-à-tête* about trying.

Before my father's mitral valve surgery, he and I had a heart-wrenching conversation about wills, wishes, requests, and documents that covered all the necessary What-Ifs that come with a parent heading into a serious operation. I felt both grown-up and six-years-old at the same time. My father handed me a list of names and phone numbers then diffused the tension with dark humor and athletic philosophy.

"These are the people I want you to call if I DNF the operation," he said. "Remember, when it comes to living, it is always better to DNF than DNS." This time, my tears fell mostly as laughter. Only an athlete would think that way, that life isn't about whether you "do not finish" your intended goal but whether you ever truly started.

The day before his procedure, my father urged me to drive the two-hour trip from his hospital in the Bronx to Philadelphia to compete with my team in the Liberty Classic. There were no Olympic points there, but I was still a pro cyclist and had a job to do with Team Colavita. My mind was still reeling from all things Olympic and aortic, but Dad and I decided a quick trip to Philly might do a mind and body good. My legs wanted to race, and so did my heart.

Our team director asked for a volunteer to "go off the front," which is cycling speak for making a solo breakaway, one of the tactics involved in saving our other teammates for the latter parts of the race. "I don't care if you DNF," our director said. "Just give it everything you have." I raised my hand, my father's words echoing within.

When it comes to living, it is always better to DNF than DNS...

For five miles, just after the start of the Liberty Classic, I broke away alone. My chances of staying away were slim to none, but for 20 minutes along Kelly Drive and the Schuylkill River, the Empress of Maybe returned. There were no thoughts of parents and mortality here, my racing mind quieted only by my racing body. Twenty beautiful minutes of Maybe. I knew the peloton would eventually catch me, and I would be gobbled up and spit out the back of its unyielding collectivity, completely shattered by exertion. The broom wagon (in the form of referees) would then sweep me into obscurity, a loose crumb fallen from the main course. But in that breakaway, my mind was silenced from all matters of disappointment, apprehension,

Olympic almostness, life, death, and hearts both literal and figurative. It was just me and my bike on a road next to a river. I was wholly in the moment of physical effort; I was neither winning nor losing, neither failing nor succeeding. I was striving and doing and seeing and feeling; I was obliterating What-Ifs and reveling in Maybes. At that moment, I was in the actual heart of what it means to be an athlete: I was trying.

My father's mitral valve repair surgery was a success. I crumpled my dad's DNF call list into a ball and tossed it into the garbage. We don't need that just yet. After seven days in the hospital, he was released, a new lease on life awaiting. He and I are in the process of reassessing exactly what is next in our respective journeys. For him, it will be a while before he can get back in the pool or on the bike. Walking is the current challenge.

"Someday, I'd like to do a sprint triathlon again, but that's a long way off," he said. "Right now, I'd just like to be able to walk over to the fridge and have myself a beer." Indeed. Not every goal needs to be of Olympic proportions or come with breakaway glories. Whatever the journey—whether it is around the world or across the kitchen—it has the potential to be a valiant effort.

All that matters is we try. All that matters is we start.

BEING THERE: THE EXTRA SPECIAL WORLD CHAMPION
September 2012

ACCORDING TO MY FRIEND FELICIA, I am the 2012 road cycling world champion. Felicia cheered me on in Limburg, Holland, in my time trial and road races in September, and since then she has referred to me as champion of the world.

"Where shall we go for lunch, world champion?" she asked, to which I quickly responded, "If I'm world champion, what do you call the 39 women who finished ahead of me in the time trial and the 80-plus competitors in the road race?"

"They're world champions, too," she said, intonating *duh.*

"And Judith Arndt and Marianne Vos, the actual world champions in the time trial and road race?" I asked.

"They're the extra-special world champions," Felicia assured me. Oh, I see. Well then, I'm sure they don't mind sharing the title with me.

"Don't you get it?" Felicia said. "You were *there.* You were at the *world championships.* That's amazing."

In some ways it is amazing. Taking into account the details of getting to the world championships for the past five years, I, too, have been downright dumbfounded that I've reached the starting line of some of these events. Given

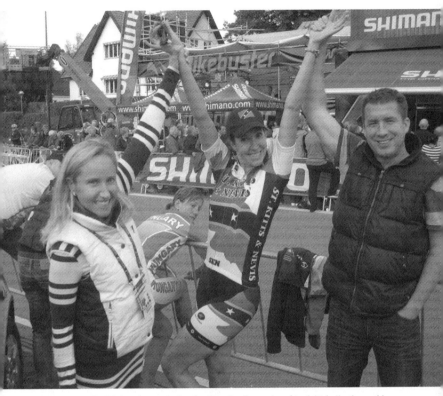

In the end, I didn't make it to the London Olympics. But my best friend thinks I'm the world champion. Maybe that's enough.

the foreign language barriers, homestay dynamics, registration protocols, and mechanical issues with my bike—all of which I often had to navigate solo—the race itself is usually the easiest part of the trip. The wickedly strong legs and unsmiling game faces of the greatest European cyclists have no physical or emotional effect on me, but trying to find a post-race banana has often brought me to tears. Worlds, man, it ain't easy.

The day after the road race in Holland, I opened an email from an anonymous sender who didn't exactly share Felicia's opinion that I should be allotted any sense of world championshipism. Since I'd finished 40th in the time trial and been broomwagoned on the sixth of eight laps in the road race (I was hardly alone—only 80-of-132 riders finished the race), the author of the email felt compelled to articulate my unworthiness. I was a complete loser. I was an embarrassment to my country. I was undeserving of being there at the world championships. Before sending the email into the trash, I had three gut reactions. My first thought was about the unknown writer himself: have we dated? My second emotion was about the ridiculousness of it all: one must be incredibly bored or angry or have severe mommy issues. Really, who sends hate mail to female cyclists? My third thought lingered on the words "being there." Even if a competitor is highly unlikely to win the world championships, does she truly deserve to be there?

I believe the answer is yes.

It is no secret that sports fans and athletes usually come in two varieties: those who believe winning isn't everything and participation is the true beauty of sports, and those who follow the Ricky Bobby philosophy of, "If you ain't first, yer last!" Yet in a sport like cycling, where there are a couple hundred competitors in the elite fields, "being there" is just how it's gonna go for about 199 of us. Not coming in first doesn't make a cyclist a loser, it makes her the majority.

On a personal level, the first time I went to the world championships in 2008 for St. Kitts and Nevis (for whom I still proudly race), the journey was about seeing how I stacked up to the best in the world. I learned I had enough talent to be there but likely not enough to be a true medal contender. Then, over the past few years as I gained political and social awareness of the subculture of professional women's cycling, I came to understand that "being there" at world championships meant a lot more than winning or losing.

Right now, women's cycling is in a tough predicament. Development programs are popping up across the world, but few if any are geared toward women and girls. While we celebrate Title IX's 40th birthday in the U.S., it's important to remember there are a lot of sports worldwide that still suffer inequality. Now more than ever it is imperative that every country granted a berth to the world championships (or any race, for that matter) should show up—to keep our numbers strong, to stay visual, to battle stereotypes—even if it may not win the race. We can, in time, win the war.

This year in Holland, only four nations sent individual members (i.e., not a full team of four to six women). Most of us traveled there via personal funds, accumulated airline miles, homestays, and handouts, as the cycling federations of smaller nations can't always supply such financial means. As athletes, we're physically trained to give everything we have—and sometimes that means our personal finances as well as grit and gumption. In my red, green, black, and yellow national-team kit, which I'd proudly designed and purchased myself, I hovered in the back of the peloton with Guam, Israel, and San Marino, where we are called to the start line last because our country has no ranking. Sometimes, no one notices we're there. But sometimes people notice change, no matter how small.

I received a little snippet of TV coverage in Holland, as many wondered where in the world St. Kitts and Nevis is, and what the cycling culture is like. A few days later, I got a new Twitter follower, a girl from St. Kitts who saw me at worlds and now she wants to start riding a bike. The greatest thing about "being there" is you never know who you might affect. I may not have won worlds, but for a couple seconds before I hit the barrier, I sure felt like I did.

For the first time in my cycling career, I took a true risk in the time trial. I entered a high-speed hairpin corner at a ridiculous speed of 30-plus mph, at the base of the famed 6 percent gradient of Cauberg Hill. I didn't cut the tangent correctly and subsequently fishtailed out of control and hit the metal barrier. Uninjured, I remounted the bike and started the climb from a dead stop, with multiple Dutch spectators (mostly male) using this opportunity to lend a hand and push my posterior up the hill. My time, henceforth, was not impressive. But, oh! The rush of almostness was permeable and undeniable. Nothing says "being there" more literally than impacting a metal barrier with your bike and body. *Here I am! Stuck in a barrier! Carpe diem!*

I had tried something new and the risk was worth the error, especially in this field of the best women in the world. I was *there!* The risk marked an improvement in my tactics, a betterment in my career. No one looking at the results would see my risk or commend me for taking a chance. They would only see a slower time, a mediocre speed. But I knew. I—and a bunch of drunk fans at the corner pub—knew that being there marked a punctuation in time, created a memory, and maybe even moved the sport forward half a centimeter.

As a competitive athlete, the question of how much

faster and better I can get gnaws at me as it does every cyclist. Trying to find the answer is the other reason I keep going back to worlds—I'm still getting better. I may not ever be an "extra-special world champion," but who knows? Someday there will be a cyclist from a small nation who will win worlds, so in the meantime, I'll keep showing up, barriers and all, to let her know that being there is possible.

THE BONUS WIFE
October 2013

MY HUSBAND'S FIRST WIFE is smiling at me from across the room. She is vibrant, beautiful, barely 30. Dressed in hiking clothes and Teva sandals, sporting cropped auburn hair and a shy grin, Colleen is waving. But not to me. This is a photograph I'm seeing, as it scrolls by slowly on our Apple TV screensaver. Colleen died nearly four years ago. Yet she visits sometimes in digital immortality where a computerized photo montage blends all of our pasts together; house cats, wedding shots, bicycle races, vacations, remission. I don't mind the old photographs, slowly floating by in their quiet juxtaposition of stillness and movement. I find them comforting. The past and the present overlap, and Colleen comes and goes. Sometimes she waves. George and I call these "winks." We wave back.

o o o

I have two separate answers when people ask me how I met my husband. Both are true, but one is simpler. The short answer is George and I met through the cycling community in Tucson, Arizona, where we both race bicycles. The longer answer goes something like this: George and I started dating seven weeks after his first wife passed away from cancer, and we married a year later. I've since learned this version doesn't fly so well when chit-chatting with a vaguely acquainted colleague in the chips and salsa aisle at Trader Joe's. Hence, the diluted answer to how we met is slightly more digestible. Or so I thought. Eventually the question, "Why?" began its circuitous dance through my mind, begging me to figure out why death, grief, love, and happiness were ingredients most people weren't willing to mix together. The answer, it turns out, is that our society may not always have the right recipe when it comes to understanding life.

I knew George and Colleen for a number of years, as we had many common friends in the cycling community of southern Arizona. From races to dinner parties, we mingled at the same events, and while Colleen and I didn't know one another too well, we were connected through the bond of shared interests and lifestyles. She was a quiet but passionate woman who practiced law for a corporate litigation firm in Tucson and spent her free time rescuing stray cats and dogs and donating to the Humane Society. Everyone liked Colleen, and her shy demeanor yet sharp determination endeared her to people. She also rode for a local cycling club and made it to the elite rank of Category 2 before the news came.

Colleen was diagnosed with breast cancer at the terribly young age of 26, just one month before she and George married in 2005. While attending law school, she defeated the first diagnosis, and the cancer went into remission. In 2007, as budding Category 3 racers, Colleen and I competed in local bike races and she became a symbol of strength and hope throughout our athletic community. I have a picture of us from the Tucson Bicycle Classic where she stands atop the road race podium wearing gold, and I stand on the second tier, a silver medal around my neck. I remember being less than pleased that the chick in remission from cancer just beat me soundly. But also profoundly proud.

In late 2008, Colleen's cancer came back with ruthless aggression, attacking her internal organs. Lesions, weight loss, and exhaustion soon followed. When the metastatic diagnosis was given, Colleen continued to fight even though it was unavoidable that the disease, now in stage IV, would take her life. The question of when, however, was still unknown. Some people live for many years with a metastatic diagnosis. But Colleen's second round of cancer proved too aggressive. She passed away October 4, 2009, in Bellingham, Washington, where she and George traveled from Tucson so Colleen could live out her last days in her childhood home among her extended family. George returned home to Arizona a few days later. Friends and family looked out for him, bringing over food for both George and the five cats Colleen had rescued from a dusty desert wash a few years before. We all struggled with the question, *What do you do for a 37-year-old guy who just lost his wife?* Like the rest of our friends, I reached out to George, asking if he wanted to get out and go for a bike ride sometime. Whenever. No rush to respond.

A few weeks later George took me up on the offer. It was good to get outside, he said. We rode, had a cup of tea, and said we'd go again sometime. We did, the next week. And the next. During our rides, we talked. Some conversations were the simple kind, where I learned about his days in the navy and his arrival in Arizona from his native New Jersey. Other times we went deeper, talking about the effects of chemo or what it's like to cook dinner for one. Sometimes George was funny.

"I realize," he said to me after a few bike rides, "that I am now a single man with five cats. I don't know what else I can possibly say about that." I assured him there was a difference between a man who helps save five strays as opposed to a man who goes to a pet store and buys five cats in one day. Besides, being a single woman with absolutely no living entities in her home, I was probably just as strange. And so our friendship began to grow. Quickly.

Within months of Colleen's passing, and after mutual examination as to how this could be possible so fast, George and I understood we were in love. Neither of us sought it out, but all of a sudden it was there. One of the reasons George and I were able to develop so swiftly through our dating relationship is that he's an excellent communicator. And I, a journalist of 15 years, like to ask questions. Combine the two and—shazam—the need for second guessing or silently wondering what the other person is thinking flies out the window. Sometimes we had deep, meaningful conversations about life and death that lasted hours into the night. We talked about life, death, marriage, love. We talked about Colleen. We talked about us. Other days we had short, easy dialogue no deeper than a puddle. Not everything had to be dissected and analyzed, and our communication was a healthy blend of serious and not.

In the last few months of her life, Colleen told George she wanted him to find love and be happy again. George said hearing those words felt like getting kicked in the chest and that being forced to consider the future was unthinkable when the present itself was barely fathomable. Yet the searing pain of her request eventually became an emotional endowment of permission, a bypass not through grief but guilt.

"After Colleen passed," George told me, "her words proved to be a beautiful gift in knowing she would have been okay with the two of us finding love." There would be no What-Ifs of the psyche, no wondering if it was okay to move forward and love again. Eight months later, George and I were engaged. He pulled a ring from his cycling jersey at mile marker 17 on Mount Lemmon where we stopped at a scenic overlook to which I paid no attention, certain that we pulled over because he must have gotten a flat tire.

I recall saying, "Oh, shit!" first, and "Yes!" second.

After all George had experienced in the throes of cancer, life, and marriage, I wanted to set the bar straight about my beliefs on love and happiness and the unknown future, just as Colleen did. I decided to share my thoughts with George via my favorite method of communication: the endurance-based run-on sentence. Passionate, raw, and slightly athletic.

"I was thinking about your conversation with Colleen about being happy and living life to the fullest so I want you to know right here and now that if I suddenly keel over tomorrow I want you to remarry wife No. 3 and be happy again and I don't care whether it is within a year or if it takes longer but make sure you put yourself out there because life is much better when you have someone to go through it with so I'm cool with all that, okay?"

"Okay. You too. Wanna go for a bike ride?"

"Yeah."

o o o

Some people—both friends and strangers—thought our togetherness was a complete lack of respect for Colleen and that George should be in mourning for a set number of years before finding happiness at "an appropriate time." We did our best to respect the variety of feelings that came our way from shock, to joy, to the whispers that ran through our circles of acquaintances. We understood that some of our friends were still mourning Colleen, and to see George with someone new was indeed an emotionally difficult situation. I told myself to grow a thick skin but was shaken at how difficult it was when judgments of disapproval were passed so easily.

From "rebound fling" to "whoring gold digger," sharp comments from friends and acquaintances circulated in a current I had little control over. No matter how painful the remarks (or inaccurate, as our middle class existence is hardly the bullseye of a gold digger's target), I knew such words came from places of anger, sadness, the frustration of grief, and the temporary release found in blame. My choice was either to feel the pain or to search for its source. Fascination, it seems, is the way my mind chooses to cauterize emotional wounds. While some comments from our friends—both those closest to us and those in the cheap seats of friendship—stung me, I did what I usually do with pain. I became its student, poking and prodding its clout until I understood where the words truly came from.

And like most lessons worth learning, so too came the buried treasures of mourning, as grief cannot exist without its predecessors: love, joy, and happiness. The quest to understand the boundaries of grief and mourning took me on a journey that was, quite frankly, not mine to begin with. Being the next love of a widower isn't easy. *That's to be expected,* people told us. But where, I wondered, did those expectations originate? Why did that lady in Trader Joe's look as though I had fed her tainted salsa instead of a love story?

The answer to our culturally acceptable traditions of mourning depends on who you ask. And if you ask History about mourning etiquette, there are some disturbing answers about the proper way to grieve. Egyptian nobility had a unique way to curb the sadness of a mourning spouse by simply burying them alive with their deceased loved one. The suttee tradition in India, until very recently outlawed, called for widows to throw themselves on the burning funeral pyres of their dead husbands. Shakespeare also gave us the slightly unhealthy notion that suicide, for a mourning young lover, is romantic. (Thanks a lot for that, Will.) But it was Queen Victoria who really set the Anti-Happy ball rolling when she decreed widows withdraw from society for two mute, black-clad years. Sure, wearing black and refusing to speak was a physically better alternative than tackling a funeral pyre, but the long-term mental repercussions of society's laws of grief may have been worse than death. No wonder we've got some messed-up roots in the grieving department.

The further I dug into the history of grief, mourning, loss, and love, the clearer it became as to how we—as present-day Americans—have become so conflicted, not just with death but with life and happiness. From the history of mourning to how we currently deal with grief (or more accurately how we often *don't* deal with it), few are the examples where hope, strength, and love get to show their place in the equation of healing. I understood then that this journey would be a new and possibly painful road for me at times.

o o o

The Christmas after George and I were married, we attended the holiday party of a colleague. I usually steered clear of in-depth conversations about how George and I met, as the timing still made some people uncomfortable. But the wife of a mutual friend pulled me aside, telling me how she was so happy George and I found each other. She sought me out to share a story about her mother passing away and the remarriage of her father.

"I was a grown woman, and I appreciated that my dad found someone new to love who was a good, kind person," the woman, CJ, explained. "I was in my forties so I didn't want to call her my stepmother, and yet it seemed too impersonal to say 'my father's second wife.' So my sister and I started calling her 'The Bonus Wife.' We meant it in the best possible way, as she saved my dad from being alone and unhappy. She was such a bonus to our family. That's what you are, Kathryn! The bonus wife. And it's a really great thing." I hugged CJ and adopted the title for my own. George enjoyed the moniker, unable to resist joking, "It sounds like I won you at a carnival." Indeed. But since life is often a three-ring circus, maybe that's accurate. I don't mind being a prize.

There's a saying about remarriage after death: women remarry, men replace. Studies show that most widows remarry an average of four years after the death of their husbands, but widowers "replace" their spouses with another in an average of two year's time. Either way, perhaps it is the perspective on replacement that needs adjusting. I agree—technically, I have replaced the role of a lost wife. *Roles* are replaceable. *People*, of course, are not. This line gets blurred too easily, as grief is anything but clear. Unless, perhaps, we change our perspective to see that role replacement can be a beautiful thing.

Four years later, the hubbub of our togetherness ceases to bring cruel words, though I have no doubt there will be some who never fully accept us. George and I navigate this particular road less traveled the best we know how—by simply following it. Sometimes it's a cerebral path, sometimes it's an actual bike lane shared on a morning ride together. Most of the time, we just let it be and see what happens. The real bonus is the present, as hard as it is to remember sometimes. Cycling remains a great reminder of living in the moment and the beauty of uncharted roads and paths unknown through the simplest of actions: riding a bike literally necessitates the action of a life moving forward. It's one of the few metaphorical loopholes where we get to remain present and move forward all at once—the ultimate bonus of a road less taken.

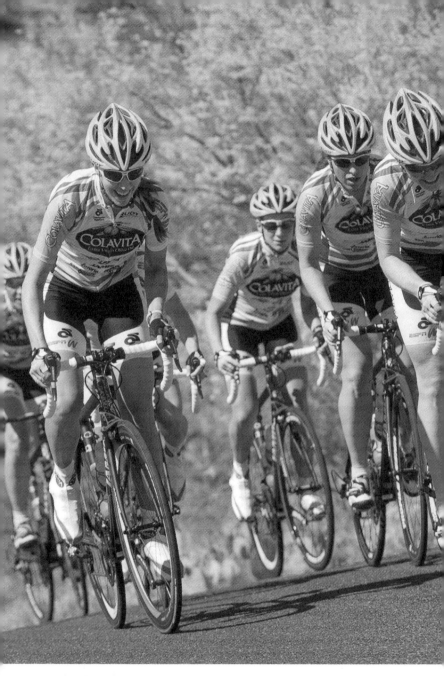

The Colavita-espnW Pro Cycling Team takes to the hills of Tucson. Among them is a rookie pro learning how to merge a career in sports, journalism, and general weirdness. (Jonathan Devich/epicimages.us)

PART IV:
MERGE

Throughout my cycling journey, I wrote for ESPN, espnW, and *VeloNews*, sometimes employed to write personal essays, other times to take a straight journalism approach to the happenings in our sport. In this section are a few of the pieces from those publications that remain close to my heart and serve as personal reminders that we are all capable of capturing a moment and sometimes using it to help create change.

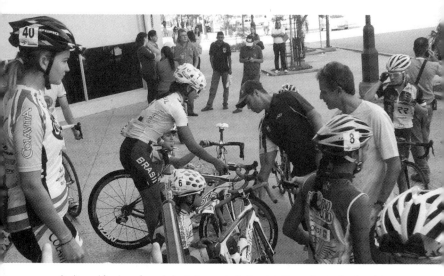

Reality and freedom of speech don't always mix. But here's to those who stand up for what they believe.

BRAZILIAN CYCLING FEDERATION TAKES A STEP BACKWARD

December 10, 2012, *VeloNews*

A COUPLE YEARS AGO, I was at the Pan-American Champion-ships in South America. I traveled alone, as I often do, as my federation's cycling budget is limited. I bring what I need with me, from spare tubes to extra tires to food and fuel. But sometimes things happen. A floor pump breaks, tubes run out, and mechanical woes lurk in the shadows, waiting to unravel a carefully constructed race plan. At this particular race, I had a loose cassette and lacked the tools to tighten my gears. In a pre-race panic, I frantically looked for help. I found hope in Brazil.

Antonio Silvestre, the road cycling coach and manager of the Brazilian Cycling Federation, was quick to help me, despite the fact I was not only the competition but also no responsibility to him whatsoever. He was kind and supportive, and he knew that no matter who I raced for, we're all part of the same sport—in women's cycling especially, where we stick together and help one another out (when not tearing one another to pieces during an event). For the past four years, I've seen Silvestre three or four times throughout a season. Without fail, he asks how I'm doing and if there is anything I need. Now, however, there is something he needs: the support of cyclists and fans who believe in cleaning up our sport.

On October 28, Silvestre was interviewed by the Brazilian TV program *Fantastic*, which was in search of an opinion on the Lance Armstrong fallout. On camera, Silvestre agreed to what the world already knew, that yes, "There is doping [in cycling]. It's a common thing." Silvestre bravely chose this moment to remind the world that doping isn't just a problem in North American and European racing, but that it's a global epidemic in sport, even in Brazil, site of the 2016 Olympics. As a coach within the Brazilian federation who traveled abroad with the national team, Silvestre noticed the pattern of results stemming from the riders in his own country. Some Brazilian cyclists were not producing the same results abroad—referring to races where drug testing is protocol—as they were at home. Hoping to call out the problem of doping in his own country, Silvestre opened up about what he believes is going on behind closed doors. He told *Fantastic*:

"I speak as the coach of the Brazilian federation, about athletes that live a fantastic period, racing for their clubs, and when they come to the selection to race outside the country, their results diminish. Why? Because they quit training? No, much to the contrary. When they go to the selection, they train 15, 20 days. They train more, and when they come to international events, they drop [back or out]. Therefore, what do you say? Why? One word: it is doping."

Three days after the TV interview, the Brazilian Confederation of Cycling (CBC) removed Silvestre from his coaching position. The CBC stated that it had "trust and confidence" that the sport is "clean" in Brazil, despite the fact that the CBC website lists nine Brazilian riders who have been given doping citations in 2012 alone. At this time, there has been no investigation launched to take a closer look into Silvestre's concerns. Silvestre, 51, a two-time Olympian in track cycling (individual and team pursuit in 1980 and 1988) who speaks five languages, has decades of coaching experience, and is largely regarded with respect among the international peloton, has chosen not to comment on the current situation. So I will.

When an upstanding coach dares to call attention to a problem within his own federation and is subsequently fired and silenced, this isn't just an issue for Brazil. This is a problem for anyone who believes in the necessity and progression of clean sport. It's a problem for all of us who believe no matter how ugly doping is, there is still hope we can clean up the mess. When the Lance Armstrong cloud broke last month, many of us clung to the silver lining that maybe now—despite the heartbreak of fallen heroes—we can rebuild the sport to a better level. Silvestre opened a door to help us get to that level by choosing to speak out on doping instead of remaining silent. Brazil slammed the door not just in his face, but in all of ours.

No matter the cover-ups and controversies that currently plague cycling, now more than ever we must remember there are good, honest people at the core of our sport who are working to amend and transform problems into solutions. They should be heard, not fired.

In a few months, my competition calendar will find me at UCI races in Central America, taking on the hills of Costa Rica and El Salvador. I'll probably lose a spare part or an energy gel, and chances are I, or some other racer, will need a little bit of help. At some point, we all need a little bit of support. Despite my wavering faith in Brazil's federation, I still have hope that Silvestre will be back at the races, wearing the colors of a trade team or national federation that believes in clean sport, sincerity, integrity, and change.

TOUR OF UTAH: HOW "MEN-ONLY" STAGE RACES HOLD BACK THE ENTIRE SPORT OF CYCLING

June 26, 2013, *VeloNews*

WHEN 13-YEAR PRO CYCLING veteran Nichole Wangsgard got a phone call to join the 2013 Tour of Utah's planning committee, her answer was an immediate yes. For Wangsgard, who currently serves as director for the Primal women's team and is a tenured professor at Southern Utah University in Cedar City, supporting the advancement of cycling is a natural inclination.

"When I got the call to help the Larry H. Miller Tour of Utah with their logistics and planning, I said, 'Yeah, sure!'" Wangsgard told *VeloNews*. "My role was to build a curriculum for the local public schools, so students and teachers could understand the sport. I got pretty excited about that." That was, until Wangsgard thought through the inevitable questions she would field, specifically, "When will you race?" As Cedar City's only professional cyclist, Wangsgard saw the obvious problem.

"Here I was, about to go tell all these kids and teachers about the joys of cycling and how fantastic the Tour of Utah is, but when they ask when I'm racing, I'll have to tell them

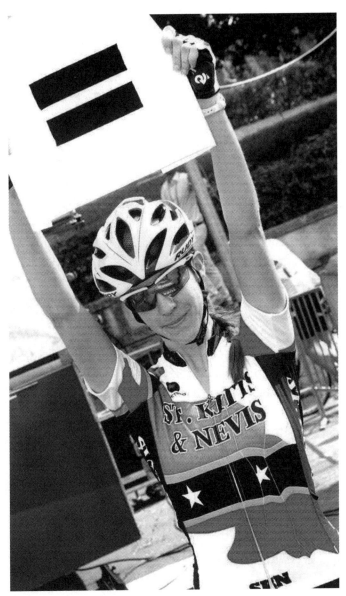

Men's stage races are great. But where are the women? (Flaviano Ossala)

I can't," she said. There is no women's professional field at the Tour of Utah. After careful consideration, Wangsgard turned down the committee position. The only question worse than, "When will you be racing?" for female pro cyclists is the subsequent question of, "Why not?"

"It just didn't sit well with me, having to tell young children that women aren't allowed in the race," Wangsgard said. "It's great that 150 of the best pro men come through town, but it simultaneously sends the message that women are not allowed to do this event."

The absence of a women's pro field in the six-day Utah tour and other men's-only stage races leads to a bigger question—are men's-only stage races hurting the growth of cycling for both genders?

The Tour of Utah is one of five UCI-sanctioned men's stage races in the United States that fail to include a UCI professional women's multi-day event. The Amgen Tour of California and the USA Pro Challenge in Colorado follow suit and are nationally televised. (Silver City's Tour of the Gila and the Tour of Elk Grove—which are not televised—do hold women's pro races, though the women's events are not UCI-sanctioned.) While the Amgen Tour does hold a single-day, invitation-only time trial event, for years female pro cyclists have lobbied unsuccessfully for a multi-day event to run in conjunction with the biggest men's tour in North America.

According to Wangsgard, the chicken-and-egg issue of adding women's races to the men's UCI events and/or the National Racing Calendar often gets caught in an unproductive blame game.

"Race directors often say they can't find enough sponsorship to hold a simultaneous women's event, while sponsors are largely unaware that women want the opportunity to race these events," Wangsgard said. "So what comes first, the media exposure, the sponsorship, or the general knowledge that women can—and want to—race these events?"

A NO-BRAINER

The majority of U.S. race directors already possess this "general knowledge" when it comes to understanding the desire women have to be included at the highest level. In the U.S. there are six NRC stage races for professional women—Redlands Bicycle Classic, Joe Martin Stage Race, Nature Valley Grand Prix, Tour of the Gila, Tour of Elk Grove, and Cascade Cycling Classic—and these race directors wonder why the men's-only races like USA Pro Challenge and Tour of Utah haven't caught on.

"Including the pro women in major stage races should be a no-brainer," said Jack Brennan, race director of the Tour of the Gila, a notoriously grueling five-day stage race in Silver City, New Mexico, which has hosted a women's field for 25 years. "The professional women are incredible."

Brennan cites that the pro women's inclusion in the race goes far beyond the economic and sponsorship values. "Sure, there are economic benefits to having a race in a small town, but it's really about the community. Colavita Pro Cycling, for example, would bring boxes of olive oil and products to the local families. They build lasting relationships. It's wonderful. You've got to remember that the economic value of a race first starts in the community. You have to get the community and the people behind you first if you want to have a financially successful event."

Redlands Bicycle Classic marketing director Scott

Welsh agrees. For 19 years, Redlands has included a professional women's field in its four-day Southern California event.

"We're really proud of our long heritage in promoting and supporting women's cycling. It's a very important component to the overall theme of bike racing. We feel like we've benefitted as much from women's cycling as anything else we do," Welsh said. "It's great to see the variety of sponsors that the women's field brings in, and we're proud to bring recognition to those sponsors who support women's cycling. Cycling is a very competitive environment, and the women put on a fantastic show. It's absolutely first class, and they work just as hard as the guys do. We're happy to support it."

Welsh also values the long-term effect of what the pro women bring to his community. "The pro women are willing to talk to groups, to school-aged kids, to sponsors. We think it's incredibly special what these athletes give back in return," Welsh said. "Not to mention it's more than just a homestay when there's a little kid in our community who gets to say, 'An Olympic champion stayed in my house!'"

GOOD FOR ALL OF SPORT

Brennan and Welsh also concur on the economic value of including women's fields alongside the men's events.

"From the marketing angle, anytime you have a community event like ours—which is 100 percent volunteer—and we're inviting the greater community of Southern California to come and watch racing, it's smart to have the diversity of events," Welsh said. "There's no doubt to the benefits of being multi-dimensional. Hundreds of thousands of dollars is generated in revenue by more than

300 professional cyclists, teams, and managers who come to the community, and with the thousands spectators… well, let's just say our city council really embraces it. This race spurs an economic boom." Better still, the Redlands Classic and Tour of the Gila don't adhere to the chicken-and-egg conundrum of sponsorship allocation in holding simultaneous men's and women's events.

"I don't think there is a difference between attracting men's and women's sponsors," Welsh said. "In fact, there are many shared sponsors. Women bring additional sponsors, which is good for both sides of the sport. When a sponsor sees a highly competitive, talented, professional female cyclist with their logo on her back, it's good for all of sport." Race directors like Brennan also tout the professionalism of the women's field as a beneficial strategy in attracting marketing and sponsorship.

"In the women's pro peloton, there are a lot of attorneys, doctors, researchers who work and race at the same time—they are smart folks. So you've got this really educated group of athletes coming into the community and getting involved in the race, and they can do so much with that. That's the one thing I would stress to these [men's-only tours]…the resources available in the women's pro peloton is incredible."

Wangsgard agrees, citing an example from her experience racing for Colavita when the team had a men's and women's program. (The Colavita men's team is now Jamis-Hagens Berman.)

"Sometimes, if the guys' team wasn't having a great race, they were thrilled when the women's team did well because it helped alleviate the burden of getting results—which is important to a sponsor. So, if there were more

UCI-level men's races that had a women's race, there would probably be more men's teams that would sponsor more women's teams, as well. Then the sponsors get that much more visibility. It's good for everyone." For Brennan, any race not including a women's field is simply selling itself short—not to mention the growth of American cycling.

"If the Tours of California, Utah, and Colorado included a pro women's race, it would expose women's racing to the greater population, which is now more than 50 percent women, and we'd have more women and young girls looking at cycling as an activity they can do," Brennan said, noting that televised media is key to growth and awareness. "But you've got to have those big televised events. [Tours of California, Utah, and Colorado] need to put the money behind a women's pro field and push it in the media. If you factor in the pro women, we'll all benefit. We'll have more race teams, more races, more women on bikes, and a high caliber of racing. But we need the big dogs to get behind it."

DOGS AND ROOSTERS

Michael Roth, VP of communications for AEG Worldwide, the driving force behind the Amgen Tour, believes the solution to the coexistence of high-profile men's and women's stage racing begins with creative marketing. Long touted as the "biggest dog" of U.S. stage races in terms of media coverage, the Amgen Tour draws both praise and backlash over the inclusion of its women's time trial. Some feel the women's event is a good start to narrowing the equality gap, while others argue that the one-day, invite-only competition is merely a band-aid solution to giving the women their due.

"We feel we've done the right thing by getting women involved," Roth said. He feels that other races like Colorado and Utah should look to California as the starting point for change—a change that could easily include creative ways of attracting sponsors.

"If Colorado and Utah also hosted a televised time trial for pro women, it could be a series people tune in to watch…almost like *American Idol*. If Tour of Utah and USA Pro Challenge could meet our commitment, then we've got something to take to sponsors and TV stations. Then what if we got Redlands, Cascade, Gila to commit to one-day TV coverage for a women's race, too? Then we've got a platform." For Roth, holding a future women's pro Tour of California starts with the women's time trial, which he sees as the first step in breaking the chicken-and-egg cycle of women's equality in racing.

"We don't want to be the chicken or the egg," said Roth. "We're trying to be the rooster."

According to Chris Aronhalt, managing partner of Medalist Sports, the firm that secures sponsorships for major U.S. events like the Amgen Tour and operated the women's Exergy Tour in 2012, television coverage plays a crucial role in drawing partnerships.

"Our clients basically watch races like the Tour de France then call us and say, 'I want that,'" Aronhalt said, regarding the demand to replicate major European races in America. A trickle-down theory of inequality comes then from what sponsors aren't seeing: a women's race broadcast alongside the Tour de France.

The 2012 USA Pro Challenge boasted 29 hours of coverage across the NBC Sports franchise over seven days of racing. Currently, there are no nationally broadcast events for women's cycling. For Wangsgard, this is unacceptable. "With nearly 30 hours of TV time for the men, surely there is a way to factor in coverage of a women's event," she said.

"I don't think it's chauvinistic," Aronhalt countered. "It's just what the sponsors see, or in this case, what they don't see." As for whose role it is to open the eyes of sponsors to the possibility of a women's race broadcast alongside the men, Aronhalt holds fast to the notion that it's not the responsibility of one individual.

"Change has to be a group effort comprised of visionaries, race owners, men, and women. Bottom line? A women's race will add more expenses, and adding more costs gets a bad reaction from sponsors. At the end of the day, it all boils down to money."

Statistics argue that female consumerism is on the rise (currently 74.9 percent of all household budgets are controlled by women), and adding a women's field could attract more sponsors and provide a larger return of investment for promoters of the major U.S. tours. Aronhalt agrees.

"Women's racing could be an asset, a true opportunity for investors to get in at the ground level," he said. "I think it's nuts not to include a women's demographic, but it's not our decision."

Whether change starts with big dogs or new roosters, Wangsgard believes race directors and sponsors won't reach their potential until USA Cycling unleashes a new plan for equality in stage races. While challenges of equality are nothing new to the women's pro peloton, Wangsgard's dilemma calls into question the advancement of all cycling, especially within the U.S. Currently, only 13 percent of USA Cycling members are women. As U.S. pro tours continue to vie for sponsorship and opportunity, the question remains whether or not the inclusion of NRC and UCI-sanctioned men's-only tours is furthering the sport as a whole.

"One way U.S. cycling can prosper for both genders is if USA Cycling makes it mandatory for any NRC or UCI-sanctioned stage race in the States to include a women's field," Wangsgard said. "Then we'd be a part of the vision of growth as a whole. It'd be such a win-win situation." Indeed, the mandatory inclusion of women's fields by USA Cycling would be a monumental advancement for the sport, not only in financial and sponsorship gains but changing societal perceptions about equality, as well. When asked if a mandate for gender equity could be in the cards in the U.S., USA Cycling's director of communications, Bill Kellick, responded that such a move would be "fiscally irresponsible and unrealistic."

"While we encourage and support equality and are absolutely committed to that end in our owned events and national calendars," said Kellick, "to mandate equality as a condition to placing privately owned, operated, and funded events on the calendar is fiscally irresponsible and unrealistic in light of the current financial pro formas of these events."

GREAT EXPECTATIONS

"What's strange is that the cycling world has fallen behind the larger non-cycling world, in terms of progress," Wangsgard said, referring to the fact that most people in the U.S. assume women are—in this post Title IX culture—allowed to race in the same events as men. "The non-cycling crowd expects women to be at races like the

Tour of Utah, and yet the rule-makers of cycling expect us not to be. That's backward. Our sport is actually behind society's expectations."

If the starting point of change begins with knowledge, then the Tour of Utah's education has begun. The race's ninth edition will roll out in Cedar City in August, and 2013 is its third year as a UCI 2.1 men's event. Jenn Andrs, project manager for the Larry H. Miller Tour of Utah, is aware that the pro women would like a stage race alongside the men.

"We really respect that the women's riders are great professionals. It sheds a great light on how capable and strong women are to cycle and do the same things the pro men are doing," Andrs said. "For 2013, we're too far down the road for including a women's component, but we're not ruling that out in the future. We have in our plans to sit down and analyze how we would be able to potentially support a women's component in the Tour of Utah in 2014 or 2015."

For Wangsgard, the knowledge that the Tour of Utah is now aware that pro women want to race is a vital first step in a long, important climb toward furthering the entire sport of cycling.

"I live in a small, conservative town," Wangsgard said. "The ratio of men to women leaders…it's not good. When it comes to sports, that attitude is passed down and women are considered not as important. I'd like to make a difference. When you really peel back the layers, this isn't just about having a women's bike race. It goes much, much deeper."

MY FATHER, THE CHEATER

June 2010, *Fathers + Daughters + Sports* (ESPN Books)

"I CHEATED," MY FATHER SAYS, panting slightly. We are at the finish line of the 2005 Escape from Alcatraz triathlon, which my 68-year-old dad, Peter Bertine, has crossed after almost four hours of athletic effort. After swimming 1.5 miles from the famous prison island of Alcatraz to the shore of San Francisco's Crissy Field, then cycling 18 miles of the notoriously hilly city, and topping it off with an eight-mile run over streets, trails, and sand, I attribute my dad's cheating comment to temporary post-race disorientation. With perhaps just a smidgen of dementia. My father, *cheat*? This is a man who turns his head *and* shields his eyes if an opponent drops one of their Scrabble tiles on the floor. Not to mention, it is pretty difficult to cheat in a triathlon.

"How?" I laugh. "Did someone give you a ride?"

"Yes," he says.

February 1986. 4:45 AM. My father's car has a thermometer that bleeps out a crisp "ding!" when the outside temperature falls below 34 degrees. My father starts the car. The ding! is immediate. It is a bitter New York winter morning. I am eleven, and my dad is driving me to figure skating practice. For six years, until I can drive myself, he will take me to my beloved, freezing, half-outdoor Murray's Rink every day at 5:00 in the morning. He will pick me up two hours later, with a chocolate chip muffin and an ice tea from the vending machine in the rink lobby. He will watch me skate, giving me the thumbs up through the Plexiglas after each maneuver I attempt. I point upward through the Plexiglas, reminding him not to stand under the rafter with the pigeon's nest. This is our routine.

The waters of San Francisco Bay are known for three things: frigidity, rough currents, and the lore of Great White sharks; it's a delightful trilogy of complications for the bizarre tastes of an endurance athlete. On the remarkably beautiful, clear, warm June day of my father's race, sharks and water temperature are not factors. The current is another story. As is often the case with openwater events, swimmers pick out a target on shore to "sight," or help keep them in line while they swim. Sometimes it is easier to follow the swimmer who's leading, provided they are sighting correctly. When the seven competitors of my father's age group (65-69 year old men) jumped into the water among the 1,500 younger triathletes, the collective of wetsuit-clad seniors smartly swam their own pace. It wasn't until the rescue boat pulled up alongside them that my father realized no one had been sighting properly and their whole tribe had drifted so far off course that the Golden Gate Bridge was almost within grasp.

The boat picked up the seven sexagenarians, brought them back to the exact spot where they drifted off-course, and kindly re-deposited them into the water rather than disqualifying the entire age group. While the rules of triathlon have a strict "no outside assistance" policy, the race directors did not find any fault with this particular situation. Except my father, who still believes he cheated by accepting the rescue-boat ride. I console him by offering an alternative perspective.

"I don't think it's cheating if you race *more* than anyone else, Dad," I say, as we check the results. "Besides, if the finish line were in Japan, your age group would have won." He finished toward the back of the 65-69 year-olds, which is just fine with him. He gives me a sweaty hug and asks, "How was your race?"

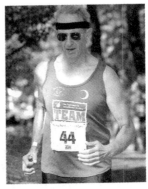

My dad, Peter Bertine, and I formed a special bond over sports.

September 1994. Freshman year of college. I am recruited to run for Colgate University. I have an argument with the coach. In the first month, she dismisses me from the team. "You should try rowing," my father says to me. Rowing is my father's sport. Every evening before dinner, the wheezy whir of his rowing machine whooshes through our home. "You'll be good at it," my father promises. "Rowing coaches usually make you run a lot, too." I mope into Colgate's rowing office, so sad about not running. The sadness soon passes. I row five-seat on the crew team during all four years of college, and under Title IX our sport is finally awarded varsity status. After graduation, I am invited to row with the U.S. National Lightweight Development team.

I finish my Escape from Alcatraz race a few hours before my father, coming in 19th in the professional women's category. There are Olympians and world champions in my field, and it is my rookie year as a pro triathlete. I am no phenom, no podium topper, no household name—just a hard-working athlete who wanted to see if it was possible to turn pro at the age of 30. Turns out it's possible. Turns out it's worth it, even if no one ever knows your name. I tell my father the details of my race, how I felt good in the water and fast on the run but that the bike felt strongest. I tell him I finished toward the back of my field, but not so bad for an old rookie.

"Like father, like daughter," my dad tells me proudly.

July 2001. Ironman Lake Placid. After three years of the short, local triathlon races I started doing in grad school, I sign up for my first Ironman event, a 2.4-mile swim, 112-mile bike, 26.2-mile marathon. Family is there to cheer me on. Dad is mesmerized, but not so much by me. "Look at all the old farts out there!" he exclaims. "Maybe I could do a triathlon." This will be his tag line for the next three years. At 66, he will sign up for his first race, the Westchester Triathlon in Rye, New York. I watch him shuffle across the finish line with his slanting lope of a stride and a huge smile on his face. I hand him Gatorade and cookies with tears streaming down my cheeks.

After our escape from Alcatraz, my father and I head to Ino's sushi restaurant in Mill Valley to celebrate our day of father-daughter athleticism. I live in Arizona, he lives in New York. Racing has kept us close in all regards. The pride of today's accomplishment is setting in, and I can literally see the experience of the day settle into his face. He has forgotten about the swim course incident. Such is the beauty of athletic achievement. Eventually, all disappointments and glitches fade away and what's left is the true reminder of why we choose to be athletes: it makes us feel alive.

"You know how I want to die?" my dad says, mid-California roll.

"I am definitely not having this conversation," I answer.

He ignores me. "No nursing home, no hospital. When I'm really old and start to lose it, I'm going to enter a triathlon.

Then, as soon as I start fading on the run, I'm going to sprint. All out. Fast as I can. None of this steady, slow, shuffling, 70-year-old stuff. I mean, I'm going to sprint until…"

"Dad…"

"…until my heart explodes! I mean, I have to go really, really fast because I don't want to half-ass it and end up in a coma or on life support, you know? I'm gonna race the life right out of me right at the very end! Woohoo! That's how you do it. You go out of this world doing what you love."

"But…"

"Don't worry, sweetheart, I'll sign a waiver."

"It won't work, Dad."

"And why is that?"

"I'd have to take your body off the course. That's outside assistance."

"No!"

"Yep. You'd be cheating."

He considers this for a moment. "Well, I guess it wouldn't be the first time."

June 2008. Vancouver, British Columbia. At the age of 72, my father qualifies for a slot at the Triathlon World Championships. I am on the sidelines cheering him on, just as he was there to cheer me on a few months ago during my Olympic trials quest in cycling. Although we're 40 years apart in age and on opposite sides of the amateur/professional ranks, my father and I are strangely indistinguishable in the world of sports. We're two old athletes with the same goal: we just want to see how far we can go, how long we can cheat the expectations of age. As my dad comes shuffling around the corner of the run course, he gives me a high-five and says, "This is my sprint lap…" I simultaneously laugh and protest. His speed never changes. He lopes off toward the finish line. This is our routine.

INVESTING IN WOMEN'S SPORTS: A PERFECT RECIPE FOR JOHN PROFACI
January 2013, espnW

IN 1978, COLAVITA, the Italian pasta and olive oil company, put down roots in the U.S., and it soon became one of the nation's top fine-foods companies. In 1999, vice president of marketing John Profaci began sponsoring a professional women's cycling team. Thirteen years later, Colavita is still going strong as one of the top-ranked U.S. cycling teams. espnW's Kathryn Bertine sat down with Profaci to discuss why investing in women's sports is smart and proactive.

Kathryn Bertine [KB]: Most sponsors are drawn to supporting a team because of a personal connection to the sport, be it as an athlete or a fan. What is your connection to cycling?

John Profaci [JP]: After graduating college in 1984, I was very fortunate to have discovered cycling, as it set me on a positive lifetime path to competitive athletics, fitness, social interaction, and outdoor travel, which I remain engaged in even 30 years later. No other physical recreation can provide so many people—no talent required—with the perfect opportunity to do "what the doctor ordered" mentally, physically, and spiritually. However, my personal preference for this activity is not the reason Colavita is a

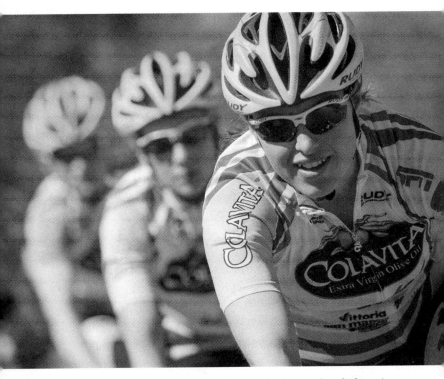

Investing in women's sports isn't just the right thing to do. It's the smart choice for financial gain. (Jonathan Devich/epicimages.us)

continuing sponsor. As marketing director of Colavita, my family and employees depend on me to spend the company money prudently. My job is to familiarize and educate home cooks around the country about our Colavita brand products. Although the "textbook" cycle of any corporate sports sponsorship is three years, I have been very pleased with the level of branding success and consumer patronage the fans of cycling have provided to Colavita. We are going on Year 13 of pro and amateur team sponsorships.

KB: As a Category 3 cyclist—which is a highly competitive field in the amateur ranks—you also own a coaching company, Full Throttle Endurance. I take it you believe sponsors should practice what they preach, so to speak?

JP: I do my best to maintain my own competitive spirit as I head into my "autumn years," and I find joy assisting other athletes, teams, and organizations with my own knowledge, contacts, and experience in sport sponsorships. After bike racing for many years, [I] decided that triathlon was the sport I would pursue personally into old age—little to no crashing there.

So with the generous and like-minded cycling-team sponsors such as Jamis Bicycles, Rudy Project, and Champion Systems, who also wish to support as many athletes as possible, I was able to assist and impact another group of men and women athletes on the Full Throttle Endurance triathlon team in New York City. This has proved to be a wonderful experience on many levels.

KB: There are many corporations that opt to back men's cycling before (if ever) considering the women's field. How did you first take an interest in women's cycling, and what kind of return on investment do you see from sponsoring women?

JP: I would say traditionally, the most effective way for a company to promote its brand in any sport has been to enter it on the men's side, simply because the media focus and attention remains skewed to the men's teams. However, because data shows that women outnumber men when it comes to household-product purchasing decisions, this creates somewhat of a dilemma for brand marketers. Unlike other corporations who sponsor only men's teams, Colavita sponsored both men's and women's team programs simultaneously. I've said this many times over the years: the reason we can support the pro men's program is because of the value we receive supporting the women's team.

KB: Tell us a little bit about how a sponsorship/partnership works when it comes to women's cycling. What needs to happen to get a cycling team off the ground?

JP: I learned about sport-team sponsorships through a NASCAR team promoter back in 1997, who pitched me on getting Colavita involved as a 10-inch-sized bumper sticker sponsor for $350,000 with one of the existing cars. Although I'm not a fan of NASCAR myself, I was intrigued by the amount of money brands were paying to get their small logo stickers anywhere on a car. Obviously, those small sponsor logos are not visible at all to spectators as the cars zoom around at 200 mph, so how can you justify the spend? Although I decided it wasn't a good fit for us, I learned that a sports sponsorship value is not necessarily about the visibility of the logo on the car—unless you are the title or a major visible sponsor—but the "license" to boast the sponsorship in your company's marketing, PR, event planning, and advertising to enchant the millions of fans of the sport. The fans of the sport embrace the brands who keep the sport alive.

A few years later, I took this marketing lesson and decided to put it in play with the more relevant sport of pro cycling for Colavita. I realized that like NASCAR, professional cycling also entertains a very loyal fan base in markets around the country who appreciate brands that sponsor their sport. The major difference is that in cycling, you can be title sponsor of a team for about the same cost as a NASCAR bumper sticker. Go figure! Sponsoring a sports team is really not all that complicated, but it takes time, a lot of money, and good staff. It's a small business with quite literally "lots of legs" to it: clothing design and production; finding equipment sponsors to help reduce costs; hiring cyclists, vehicles, insurance, staff, etc. But so many companies back away quickly from sports sponsorships because they don't realize the most important part of the sponsorship: the need to integrate the plan into the overall consumer-marketing plan to enchant the millions of fans of the sport. The return on investment cannot be justified simply by the printed logo on the clothing and cars, and so most brands come and go.

KB: Title IX recently celebrated its 40th anniversary, yet we know there is still a lot of ground to cover in terms of equality for women's sports—cycling especially, where women are not always given the same race opportunities, sponsorships, or salaries as the men. As a sponsor, what are the biggest challenges you see in women's cycling, and what can we do to overcome them?

JP: A more balanced and equal media focus between men's and women's pro cycling has come a long way in the U.S., but nowhere near what occurs in Europe. For instance, when the Giro Donne [women's Giro D'Italia] is occurring each season, you can watch that great women's-only race event in every Italian household on TV. Think about this: Western Europe fits within half of the land mass of the U.S., and there were more than 30 UCI-registered pro women's teams, as compared to only two in the U.S. during the 2012 season. The most talented U.S. women cyclists therefore need to live and race in Europe, not only because of the level of competition, but also the opportunity to earn a living with better prize money. All of those UCI pro women's teams in Europe exist because of the additional publicity provided to the women's side of the sport. As a result, more companies can invest in the sponsorships because there is actual return of investment by way of news reporting and visuals of their brand. This doesn't happen in the U.S., and unless U.S. media companies—newspapers and websites—start dedicating more time and space to women's cycling, the women's sport will never really grow here, which is a shame.

KB: The recent scandals within men's cycling have caused some sponsors to withdraw their support not just from men's cycling but from the women's peloton, as well. Do you think this reasoning is justified?

JP: I imagine there is a trickle-down theory there, but I don't think anyone who pays attention to cycling believes [cheating/doping] is happening to the same extent on the women's side. Cycling is bigger than the pro ranks. For a company or sponsor to pull out of a sport that is fun, healthy, recreational, and is something millions of people do every day…that shouldn't happen. I don't believe Lance Armstrong or anyone else involved in scandal can take the true essence away from cycling. It might take something away from the high-level men's side of the sport, but that is not everyone's interest. I don't think Armstrong or anyone else doing something negative on the men's side is going to have a lasting impact on the women's side of cycling. I can't see a spectator watching a pro women's race and associating it with Lance Armstrong. That doesn't happen. The women are their own sport.

For Colavita, we have an audience that grows every year. My interest is local teams, pro women and amateur riders of all abilities. Companies need to remember the bigger picture when it comes to sponsorship. They can't just sit back and say, "Where's my return of investment?" They have to go get the value. They have to promote and have pride in their commitment. That's the bigger part of the value of supporting sports.

KB: Colavita has had 12 Olympians, one world champion, and 12 national champions on the team during its 13-year run, which is directly related to your role in enabling these women to compete professionally. Did you ever imagine that pasta and olive oil could yield such powerful results?

JP: It's a great feeling for me to see those statistics and accomplishments of the many athletes who were part of our Colavita women's team at some point of their careers. Needless to say, I hope all of them will remember Colavita when they finish pro cycling and spend more time shopping and cooking! Ha!

But seriously, I feel very satisfied on a personal level that my decision to support this team has helped so many young women athletes over the years. That satisfaction has nothing to do with the business return.

COLAVITA'S ATHLETE HALL OF FAME
OLYMPIANS

Iona Wynter Parks (Jamaica), Rachel Heal (U.K.), Dotsie Bausch (U.S.), Giorgia Bronzini (Italy), Jasmin Glaesser (Canada), Sue Palmer-Komar (Canada), Rushlee Buchanan (New Zealand), Cath Cheatley (New Zealand), Modesta Vžesniauskaitė (Lithuania), Kate Bates (Australia), Sarah Ulmer (New Zealand), Melissa Holt (New Zealand)

WORLD CHAMPION
Giorgia Bronzini, Italy—road race (2010, 2011)

NATIONAL CHAMPIONS
U.S.
Tina Pic—criterium (record six national titles)
Theresa Cliff-Ryan—criterium (2011, 2012)
Alison Powers—time trial (2008)
Jessica Phillips—time trial (2009)

CANADA
Sue Palmer-Komar—time trial (2004, 2005), road race (1996)
Leah Kirchmann—criterium (2011)

NEW ZEALAND
Cath Cheatley—road race (2011)
Rushlee Buchanan—criterium (2010)
Melissa Holt—road race and time trial (2001, 2008, 2009, 2010)

AUSTRALIA
Kate Bates—road race (2008)

ST. KITTS and NEVIS
Kathryn Bertine—road race and time trial (2009–12)

SKIRTING THE ISSUE: BOXING'S STEP BACKWARD

November 2011, espnW

LAST WEEK, THE STORY BROKE about the Amateur International Boxing Association (AIBA) asking its female competitors to abide by a new dress code. The AIBA called for the women of boxing to drop traditional knee-length shorts and don skirts inside the ring.

The reason? The AIBA believes it will help spectators distinguish women from men. That, and as Polish coach Leszek Piotrowski, who made the skirt suggestion mandatory for the Polish team, put it: "By wearing skirts, in my opinion, it gives a good impression, a womanly impression. Wearing shorts is not a good way for women boxers to dress."

Huh. I had no idea boxing was beguiled by such a predicament. Let's see if we can come up with a solution. For starters, we can always use our eyeballs to aid in differentiating men from women. Should that prove complicated, written words are helpful, as in labeling tickets and TV banners with "Women's Boxing." If those fail, there's the tried-and-true method of simply not caring about gender and choosing to watch boxing—or any sport—because of the competition. But skirts? We already have an organized event showcasing female fighters in skirts. It's called middle school. Time to grow up, AIBA. Let women choose what they want to wear.

Here we are on the eve of the 40th anniversary of Title IX, and we're still fighting goofy clauses that threaten to set female athletes back decades in our quest for equality. We should be making great strides in everything from salaries to women's professional leagues to introducing little girls into the realms of male-dominated sports. Instead, thanks to organizations like AIBA, we're dealing with inseam regulations.

Skirts have been around in women's sports since the beginning of time—or at least since 1900, if we go by the inclusion of female athletes at the Paris Olympics. Tennis, field hockey, figure skating—skirts are the norm in many athletic venues. The difference is that these sports and athletes are choosing to uphold tradition. No one is making the participants wear skirts. Uh-oh...participants. That's not very feminine. I mean particiskirts.

Even modern sports like triathlon and recreational running have women competing in athletically engineered skirts, giving ladies the opportunity to look cute and sassy while they race and work out. Some women love the skirts. Personally, it throws me off when I see a woman running in a skirt. My reaction is to wonder who's chasing her. Someone with a weapon? Maybe a briefcase? Still, these skirts are a choice, not a rule.

As for the boxers at the heart of the debate, the female fighters seem to be in agreement about the absurdity of the regulation, according to an interview by the BBC.

"It's a disgrace that they're forcing some of the women to wear those miniskirts. We should be able to wear shorts, just like the men," said Katie Taylor, a three-time world champion from Ireland.

"It should be the boxer's choice whether they want to or not. You shouldn't be forced to wear one," British lightweight champion Natasha Jonas said.

On one hand, the issue is amusing in its datedness. On the other hand, it's pretty frightening. The message boxing is sending to the world is this—women's sports are all about looks, not athleticism. On top of that, AIBA isn't listening to what its athletes want and need. When an athletic institution isn't looking out for its players' best interests, it's a blow to athletes in every sport.

If we let the AIBA force skirts in boxing, we might as well endorse wardrobe changes in other women's sports.

Let's make tiaras mandatory for female cyclists. Those silly helmets just don't bring out their eyes. And bikinis for platform divers. Such great bodies, why not add a risqué element by combining high-impact speed with halter tops? That's a 10.0, baby. How about hot pants for equestrians? Chaps are so, like, 1832. And just to be safe, filed épée tips for women's fencing. Really, women shouldn't be running around with sharp objects—unless they're in the kitchen, of course.

My choice for settling the matter of the boxing's uniform woes would be to have the skirt-suggesting member of the AIBA step into the ring with one of its athletes. The AIBA representative can wear the skirt, the athlete can wear the shorts, and whoever wins gets to enforce the dress code. Seems fair. But when it comes to mixing female athletes with media-generating publicity stunts, fair isn't usually part of the equation. Lady boxers of the world, keep fighting until it is. Your fellow female athletes are behind you. We look forward to women's boxing making its debut next year at the London Olympics. By then, we hope the focus is on your fists and not your hemlines.

I plan to be there in my tiara, cheering you on.

ADONAL FOYLE TEACHES GROWL POWER
July 2011, espnW

ON A HUMID SUMMER DAY on the Caribbean island of Dominica, 1,400 miles south of Miami, two men with rusted machetes quietly crossed an outdoor basketball court populated with young children. The children paid the knife-wielding trespassers no mind. The men were on their way to work in the rain forests, their long blades used for making trails and felling fruit from trees. The kids were more captivated by the white bus pulling up to the basketball court. Sixteen coaches and volunteers emerged, one standing 6'10" with a towering physique of muscle and power. A young boy approached the enormous man, who wore the long shorts and cutoff sleeves synonymous with basketball garb.

"Are you Shaq?" the boy asked.

Adonal Foyle leaned down to the child, feigning great offense.

"I am *much* prettier than Shaq," he said. The child laughed and ran away from the gentle giant.

Foyle, who retired in 2010 after a 12-year NBA career, surveyed the new basketball court, set into a hillside in rural Grand Fond, Dominica. Last year his foundation refurbished the court with fresh pavement, paint, backboards, and hoops. "We're going to have a lot of campers today," he said. "Let's get ready."

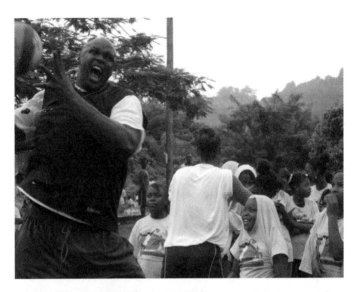

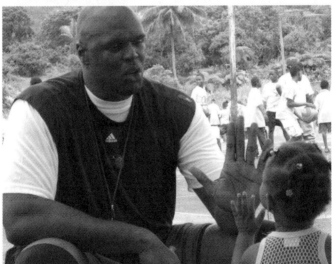

Thirteen-year NBA veteran (and my old college buddy!) Adonal Foyle demonstrates how including girls in sports can lead to great futures for everyone.

Boxes of basketballs, T-shirts, water bottles, children's books, nutritional pamphlets, and bright orange Gatorade jugs were unloaded from the bus. Besides the boxes and containers and sporting equipment, the volunteers also unpacked the deeper messages of Adonal Foyle's Athletics & Academics Island Youth Camps: hope, equality, and betterment, a trilogy of life lessons with which Foyle is extremely familiar.

The story of Adonal Foyle seems to be the stuff of a Disney screenwriting project. In 1990, two professors from Colgate University in Hamilton, New York, Jay and Joan Mandel, were in the Caribbean doing research. They saw a 16-year-old standing almost 7' tall, playing in a basketball camp. He barely knew how to dribble. The kid came from the island of Canouan in St. Vincent and the Grenadines, where his family had to light their home with only one kerosene lamp. The Mandels recognized the boy's potential. Within two weeks, Foyle was living with them in the United States and attending public high school. Reading and writing at the level of his peers was a challenge for Foyle, who worked tirelessly on his vocabulary and his studies. His drive and determination to learn thrived in upstate New York, and so did his basketball skills.

Foyle led his Hamilton Central High School basketball team to a 1994 state championship. That spring, he stunned the recruiters of Duke, Syracuse, and just about every other basketball powerhouse by choosing to stay local. He enrolled at Colgate, which has a small but feisty Division I basketball program in the Patriot League. Foyle brought the Raiders to the NCAAs in 1995 and 1996, where they fell to Kansas and Connecticut, respectively. At the end of his junior year in 1997, the Golden State Warriors took Foyle as the eighth pick in the NBA draft. He spent 10 years with Golden State before heading to the Orlando Magic for the final two years of his career. (There was a brief, one-month stint with the Memphis Grizzlies, but he re-signed with the Magic after Memphis waived him.)

Foyle averaged 4.1 points and 1.6 blocks per game in his career, and he finished in the top 10 in the league in blocks four times. Aware of education's value, Foyle continued his studies while on the road and graduated from Colgate in 1999 with a degree in history. He is currently finishing work on a master's in sports psychology at John F. Kennedy University in California and believes that a doctorate is in his future.

Off the court, Foyle, 36, runs two charities: Democracy Matters, which encourages college students to get involved with politics; and the Kerosene Lamp Foundation, named for the beacon of light in Foyle's youth, which provides support and incentives for kids to succeed in school. The KLF funds Foyle's summer camps and essay competitions and refurbishes neglected basketball courts in the U.S. and in the Caribbean islands.

Not bad for a kid from a tiny Caribbean island without cars and a home without electricity. Some believe Foyle will someday serve as the president of Canouan. But for now, Foyle is happiest when he's teaching little girls how to snarl.

At the Dominica camp, more than 130 kids ages 5 to 17 were bused in from nearby villages on the island, which has a population of 72,000. The youngsters were divided among the volunteers, who included professional coaches, college players, and teenagers from the U.S. spending their summer vacation helping others. Foyle also chose three teenagers from the island of St. Vincent to work for the camp, a reward for both their basketball and academic prowess. After all, it was here on Dominica that Foyle himself was discovered 21 years ago. But while no NBA scouts (or well-intentioned college professors) observed the day's camp, Foyle is aware that his efforts to give back are moving things forward in the Caribbean. This camp marked a positive turn as more female athletes attended it than in the seven-year history of his camps.

Foyle rotated through the groups, overseeing the drills and techniques. A bunch of young ladies did drills with volunteer Jamila Veasley, who played basketball at UCLA. Foyle snatched up a ball and showed a swarm of preteen girls how to rebound.

"It's pretty to growl," Foyle insisted loudly. The key is having the confidence, quickness, and fight to go after the ball, he told the girls. Putting on his game face, Foyle demonstrated, letting loose a monstrous battle cry and ferocious look while charging to the hoop to collect a rebound. The girls giggled, realizing Foyle is a gentle soul. Beneath his growl, they sensed that he was teaching them a bigger lesson: *Go after what you want.*

o o o

What Foyle wants is twofold: to give the kids of the Caribbean a leg up in life by touting the lessons of sports and academics. "You have to have this duality between sports and academics," Foyle said. "When we first started the camp, we wanted to find a way to connect basketball and academics. If you look at the logo of our T-shirts, it's a basketball in one hand and a book in the other. That's the metaphor and symbolism for what we are trying to do, which is to blend the athletic discipline with the schooling discipline for a life well-lived."

Fun as the camp may be, Foyle doesn't let the education factor slip past his campers. During a water break, he asked his crowd of kids what they thought the average number of career years for an NBA player was. Hands shot up. "Ten! Twelve! Fifteen years!" the kids shouted. Foyle enunciated the reality slowly: 3.7 years. He didn't mention that his career was nearly four times as long. Instead, he emphasized the importance of education, telling the kids that at the end of camp, everyone would receive books. Only some would get basketballs.

"I think that in the U.S.—and a lot of other places—we forget that a lot of these kids aren't going to make the NBA. We have to give them the opportunity to become well-adjusted and well-educated adults," Foyle said. The heart of his camp revolves around opportunity, which doesn't come easily in Third World nations during a global economic meltdown. While cricket, soccer, and track top the ranks of popular sports in most Caribbean nations, basketball is still relatively new. But NBA stars such as Patrick Ewing (Jamaica) and Tim Duncan (St. Croix) originally hailed from the islands, and Foyle believes the Caribbean has big potential in basketball. "We have all these big, tall guys," he joked.

Because athletics without an education doesn't mean much in the long run, Foyle provides the opportunity for both and leads by example. "When you work with young people, you have to walk the walk as well as talk the talk," said Foyle, who continues to walk the walk as the Magic's director of player development during the NBA's regular season. In the summer, he hits the islands with his camps, preaching the good word of sports and education with emphasis on the latter.

"I believe that knowledge is who we are ultimately," he said. "When the ball is laid to rest, and everything is done, we always rely on knowledge. I'll be happy if we [the Caribbean] have some NBA players, but I'll be very ecstatic if we have some great college players and some great kids who go to college."

For players from smaller countries with fewer opportunities, college hoops and the NBA are icing on the cake, but Foyle knows opportunity is the prime ingredient for change and development.

"I don't want everybody to play basketball," he said. "I want everybody to have the *opportunity* to play basketball to figure out what they like."

As for the girls of Dominica, they seem to have figured out they like basketball very much. The number of female participants has doubled from last season's camp, giving Foyle a bright outlook on the future of Caribbean women in sports.

"It is very important to empower young ladies to grow into very well-educated adults. We have had more females in our camp because we make it more accessible to them. We want them to come, we encourage them to come… and most of the time, they are much better shooters than the boys," Foyle said. He added with a laugh: "We tell the boys, 'Get up to the standard of the ladies.'"

The secrets of a growling rebound cross into everyday life lessons for Foyle's young female campers. Being an athlete is an education in sociology, one that girls often desperately need. According to Foyle, it's a great thing for a woman to be both tough and graceful. "How you merge those things is very important," he said. "[Girls] have been taught through society that it is not okay to be physical and to be aggressive. I want them to know it is okay to be aggressive. I grew up in a house with a women's studies professor, so I know it is okay to growl as a woman, and be amazing and powerful. I think the future holds great promise for girls."

THE FIRST WOMAN OF LITTLE LEAGUE: KATHRYN "TUBBY" JOHNSTON
April 2011, espnW

IN THE SPRING OF 1950, Tommy Johnston did what lots of 11-year-old boys did in Corning, New York: he signed up for local Little League tryouts. His big sister, Kathryn, 12, decided to accompany him. But before they left the house, Kathryn had one request of their mother.

"I had two long braids, and I asked my mother to cut them off," she said. "I put on a pair of slacks and one of my brother's T-shirts. Then I tucked my new short hair up into a ball cap." When they arrived at the diamond, Kathryn announced to her brother that she was going to try out for the baseball team as well and then quietly stepped into the record books as the first girl to play Little League.

"My brother, Tommy, was shocked and said I couldn't play because I was a girl. But I wasn't going to let that stop me.… I was stronger than him. He was a skinny little thing," Kathryn "Tubby" Johnston Massar said, laughing, in a recent phone interview. "But my father always took me out, and we would play baseball. He would throw the ball, and I would bat. So I went out for the team." Now 73, and a resident of Yuba City, California, Johnston Massar recalls her Little League days in upstate New York as the most formative years of her childhood. But before learning the dynamics of boys' baseball, Johnston Massar first had to school herself in the craft of illusions.

Fearing that the Little League coaches wanted nothing to do with little girls, Johnston dressed up as a boy, walked over to the sign-up table, and penned the name Tubby Johnston. "I loved the Little Lulu comic books, and my favorite character was a boy named Tubby," Johnston Massar said. "Besides, I was a short little kid and hadn't started to develop. The tryouts were on the south side of town, and none of the kids there knew me, so that was helpful."

The coaches liked what they saw during tryouts and assigned "Tubby" to the Corning King's Dairy team as a lefty-throwing, righty-hitting first baseperson. "I still didn't want to tell the coaches I was a girl. I stayed disguised as a boy for almost a week, but I was awfully uncomfortable someone would find out and throw me off the team. So I finally confessed to the coach. He said, 'Well, if you're good enough to make the team, you're good enough to stay on the team.'"

Despite Tubby's proven ability as a ballplayer, not everyone approved of her presence. "There was no rule that a girl couldn't play Little League, but we certainly weren't welcome," she recalled. Parents often objected, as did coaches of opposing teams. "I think they were so upset because I was a good player and I think they thought I was showing up their sons," Johnston Massar said.

The news of Johnston's presence made its way back to Little League headquarters in Williamsport, Pennsylvania, and at the end of 1951 (when Johnston turned 13 and was no longer eligible to play Little League, which had a

12-and-under cap at the time) the Tubby Rule was handed down. Girls were not allowed to play in Little League. It was an odd juxtaposition, since the popular American Girls Professional Baseball League—the inspiration for the movie, *A League of Their Own*—had already been in existence for nearly a decade.

The Tubby Rule stood until 1972, when Maria Pepe, a 12-year-old from Hoboken, New Jersey, sued Little League for the right to play. The case went to the New Jersey Supreme Court and was backed by the National Organization for Women. The verdict came back in favor of Pepe in 1974, and girls were officially allowed into Little League.

Today, there are 2.7 million children between the ages of five and 18 registered with Little League. While the organization does not keep track of female baseball players specifically, the number of girls in baseball is rising. So, too, is their talent. In April 2009, 12-year-old pitcher Mackenzie Brown of Bayonne, New Jersey, made the record book as the first girl to throw a perfect game—she retired all 18 boys in the lineup, striking out 12.

No matter how many records are broken and titles earned by present-day girls in baseball, every female Little League player shares Tubby Johnston's sentiments. "I was just a young girl who wanted to play baseball. I loved baseball, and I didn't think being a girl should keep you from playing," Johnston Massar said.

Tubby Johnston–turned–Kathryn Massar recently retired after 32 years as a triage nurse; she still cites her Little League experience as the cornerstone of both her career in medicine and her family values. "Any sport is a form of discipline and leadership and makes you a team player," attests Johnston Massar, whose story is being developed into a movie for Disney.

As for Tommy, the little brother once embarrassed by his sister's baseball tryout, "Well, he turned out to be really proud of me," she said. "A few weeks into Little League, he left his team and joined mine. We were a great shortstop-first base combo."

BIG WHEEL
March 2005, *ESPN The Magazine*

"THERE'S A PLAYGROUND I've been checking out," Kris Holm tells me in a quiet voice. For a variety of reasons, this is not a sentence that most 32-year-old men should publicly state. But something tells me I need not fear this man. For starters, he is holding a unicycle. In addition, he's Canadian. Add the small detail that Holm is a world champion athlete and suddenly the local Vancouver playground seems like a very interesting place to go.

Holm, who stands 5'10" and sports a tousle of blond hair beneath his helmet, has the Clark Kent façade going for him. His slight build and polite manner would lead the average person to assume Holm is more likely a docile librarian than an extreme-sport athlete. There is no bravado about him, no stray piercings, no look-at-me-I'm-a-multi-colored-badass tattoos, no vocabulary of hype or slang. The man holds a master's degree in physical geography and works for an engineering firm. No one walking by would ever guess that Holm hits speeds of 40 mph traveling down mountains on a unicycle. Or that he's ridden his wheel around the lips of volcanoes, pedaled the railings of 200'-tall bridges, or even rolled along the Great Wall of China. No one would ever assume that Kris Holm might be the next Tony Hawk, Jake Burton, or Gary Fisher.

But he is. Laugh as you might about unicycling becoming mainstream—just as they laughed about surfboards on the snow—but by the end of this decade, anyone who owns a skateboard, snowboard, or mountain bike will likely make room in the garage for their *Kris Holm Unicycle.*

From a hill overlooking downtown Vancouver, a multi-colored, plastic entanglement of swings, slides, and metal ladders rises out of a playground's gravel pit. The sky threatens rain, and there is no one around. Holm is wearing battered shin guards, a silver helmet, and a crimson jersey from his clothing sponsor, Horny Toad. With no more effort than it takes to sit on a couch, Holm mounts his 15-lb. signature *Kris Holm* knobby-tire unicycle and plows a trail through the gravel. For those of us who have difficulty walking in gravel, the unicycle equivalent would be like trying to break dance in quicksand. But Holm is merely warming up. Once the man is on his unicycle, it is impossible to look away.

After a few minutes of pedaling, he grips the handle under his uni-seat and in a pogo-stick motion bounds up—*up!* – the slide's ladder, the tire boinging from rung to rung. At the top of the plastic contraption, a good 15' above ground, Holm rides the rims and railings of the entire playground structure, looking for what he calls "good lines," which is unicycle code for anything rideable. In Holm's case, that means anything larger than the width of a dime. As he prepares to jump off the piping of the monkey bars and land upright in the gravel, a small boy walking past the playground tugs on his mother's sleeve. "Mooooom!" he says, pointing toward Holm. "Look what *he's* allowed to do!" They watch Holm fling himself off the structure and land wheelfirst in the gravel. The mother hurries her son along.

THE ROAD LESS TAKEN

∘ ∘ ∘

Unicycling evolved in the mid-1800s when a British farmer named Penny Farthing removed the small rear wheel of his bicycle and discovered the big wheel held its own as he teetered about his farm. Apparently, Farthing must have been somewhat of a loner because the sport didn't catch on for another century and a half. Now there appears to be a unicycling genre for every athletic personality. Freeride mountain unicycling necessitates a mountain, lots of stumpy obstructions, and an endurance factor for the long-distance side of it. For those who wish not to one-wheel it off a cliff, there are plenty of other disciplines. Trials unicycling, which is Holm's specialty, involves riding over, on, or through any kind of obstacle, whether natural or manmade. Street unicycling is similar to the skateboard half-pipe and BMX ramps, the idea being that barriers are staged to set up tricks. For those wanting a team atmosphere, there is unicycle basketball, hockey, polo, and just about any other major league adaptation. And for the figure skater in all of us, there is artistic freestyle unicycling. Often done in a gymnasium, it shows off one's skills as music plays and sequins are worn. "I've never done that," Holm defends. While Holm has done nearly everything else on a unicycle, from encircling skyscraper roofs to slaloming through ski moguls, his introduction to the sport was hardly death-defying.

In the spring of 1986, eleven-year-old Holm saw a street performer named Yuri Toufar zipping around on a unicycle while playing a violin in downtown Vancouver. "I played the violin, too, so I thought it would be fun to try a unicycle," Holm, a Vancouver native, reasoned. His parents tracked one down and gave it to him for his 12th birthday, oblivious to the legacy they were creating. During the next 13 years, Holm hopped, swerved, mounted, and crashed his way along the driftwood and rocks that inhabited the city's shoreline. Slowly, his primary interest in rock climbing fell by the wayside, and Holm devoted all his free time to perfecting his skill level.

His original sport, however, had already given Holm an advantage. Rock climbing bequeathed to Holm a feeling of ease in precarious situations. Heights were not a problem. Neither was negotiating balance or bodily control. Mentally visualizing routes and making quick decisions came easy on a unicycle after practicing it on above-ground rock faces.

In 1998 Holm, who figured he was the only person unicycling on an everyday basis, made a startling discovery. An Internet search delivered the shocking news that Holm was not the only one in his universe. There were others out there. Numerous dotcoms, personal blogs, college clubs—hundreds of sites devoted to the single-wheel passion. "It was like finding a world I never knew existed before. For 12 years I rode in a vacuum. Just imagine what it's like to be really into a sport and not know that anyone else in the world does it, too." Inspired, Holm began to design equipment. Noting the shortage of unicycle dealers and the fact that most unicycles were pieced together from old bicycle parts, Holm envisioned a market that would cater to the advancement of the unicycle. There had to be a better way to make a mountain unicycle than wrapping twine around slick tires. There had to be something more advanced than steel hubs and soldered-on axles that needed re-soldering every three weeks. After floating his sketches and plans of a more stable, inexpensive unicycle to various companies for three long years, Holm finally found an investor.

"I went to NORCO Bikes and they very reluctantly said, 'Okay, we'll give it a shot,'" Holm said. Within a few months, Holm designed a signature line of three road and mountain unicycles. Simultaneous to Holm's unicycle manufacturing plans, the unicycling population began to grow. Unicycle.com organized a governing body, and the sport began holding regional competitions throughout the U.S. and Canada. Holm jumped on board to organize the first national unicycle trials competition, where competitors were scored on technical tricks and obstacle maneuvers. The first competition in 1999 saw 35 entrants. In 2004, there were more than three hundred. In addition to Holm's riding schedule and day job, he also manages Kris Holm Unicycles, designs equipment, and tests products. Last year, Kris Holm Unicycles grossed better than $250,000 in sales, tripling the previous year's mark. While that amount might seem like spare change to some sports markets, Holm considers it a stellar start. He acknowledges that most mainstream bike companies view mountain unicycling as an unlikely pastime, and he focuses on a positive statistic. "Unicycling's current status is very similar to mountain biking 30 years ago," Holm said, referencing sales and growing popularity. KHU is nothing if not innovative. Next year the company will debut the first *geared* mountain unicycle. Gears. On a unicycle. A hundred years ago, bicycle companies toyed with a similar idea. Currently, Kris Holm Unicycles sends hundreds of unicycles, components, and clothing to New Zealand, Europe, North America, Australia, and Japan. And while Holm fosters the global sprawl of unicycling, he sets an environmental precedent by becoming the first cycling company—regardless of wheel count—to donate 1 percent of all profits to environmental conservation.

o o o

Regarding the athleticism of unicycling, Holm weighs in on the physical benefits. He explains that there is no coasting on a unicycle as there is on a two-wheeled bike. On one wheel, the rider must pedal continuously for balance, whether traveling uphill or down. "It's a full-body workout," Holm offered, citing the uni-benefits. "Keeping your arms out to the side and pulling up the unicycle, you build good arms and shoulders as well as strong quads and hamstrings." And for the hard data, a serious mountain unicycle rider can see heart rates rise to 170 bpm. One of Holm's riding partners, Nathan Hoover, recorded his heart-rate info during a 6.2-mile race. After the 1-hour 17-minute course, Hoover hit a max heart rate of 169 bpm, averaged speeds of 5.6 mph, and gained 823' of elevation. "I'm able to race just as hard on a unicycle as I am on a bike," Hoover claimed, citing that riding a unicycle uphill (and down) is the best physical training he's ever come across. And one might take his word, seeing as Hoover and Holm unicycally conquered the 18,500' Mexican volcano, El Pico de Orizaba.

The muscular advantages of unicycling seem to be a hot new cross-training secret of some of the world's top athletes. Targeting the muscles of the abs and the lower back, unicycling requires a steady core just to mount the cycle, let alone ride it. Downhill skiing champion Bode Miller rides a unicycle. So does Hall of Fame quarterback Steve

Young, pro skateboarder Rodney "Mutt" Mullen, and former Formula One world champion Mika Hakkinen. The joy of unicycling has also found its way under the likes of actor Johnny Depp, comedian Eddie Izzard, reggae legend Peter Tosh, and even our own superfly secretary of defense, Donald "Uni Dude" Rumsfeld. According to 1970s rock-climbing pioneer John Long, mountain unicycling may be one of the best-kept training secrets in athletics. "It is exhausting," Long said, "there is no rest. Every time the wheel turns, your leg turns, and it'll cook your legs in less than 300 yards." Also, people will gawk openly at anyone who tries it.

While the unicycle has become a more publicly accepted sight in the past few decades, Holm still receives his fair share of stares and comments. Granted, the unicycle is a strange contraption. We're used to seeing wheels in multiples of two, and anything else looks, well, broken.

"There is something about seeing a unicyclist that makes people lose all self-consciousness," Holm said. "People will hang on the windows of moving cars to shout at me, asking where my other wheel is, stuff like that." But Holm remains unfazed, convinced that unicycling is no more outlandish than cycling or jogging.

"Think about it," he reasoned, comparing unicycling to mainstream sports. "Why would you throw a ball through a hoop or hit a ball with a stick? It just makes you feel good. It's fun." Hoover is quick to agree, citing that Holm has done more for the sport of unicycling than anyone else, changing it from a geekish activity to an up-and-coming sport worthy of X Games status. "Kris completely defined what is possible on a unicycle," Hoover said. "Besides being physically skilled and strong, his mental power is beyond what most people ever encounter." John Long agreed. After seeing Holm bring a unicycle on a rock-climbing trip and ride summits and ledges, Long knew he was witnessing the birth of a new sport. "No one thought about that before, combining climbing and unicycling. Kris is in another realm as far as sports go. He invented mountain unicycling, and he set the bar awfully high."

o o o

After Holm tires of the playground, we drive across town to the famous freeride mountain bike trails of the North Shore Forest outside Vancouver. Two miles into the trees (by wheel and foot), a series of bizarre manmade log obstacles copiously winds between the Redwoods. Rickety wooden ladders, seesaw planks, train-track slats, and way-too-high ramps hover over the rocky forest floor and give the impression that one has stumbled into the lair of a mutant hamster. The place is eerily quiet. Sighting an Ewok or a Yeti would be less surprising than what I am about to see. On a moss-covered log, 10' above ground and at least 30' long, Kris Holm ricochets by and launches himself off the obstacle, then wheels down the rest of the mountain we just hiked up. Two mountain bikers pull off the trail to watch Holm descend. "It's not every day you get to ride behind greatness," he said to his friend. "That's Kris Holm. The guy's insane."

Over the next two hours, Holm takes some nasty falls that would make Bam look like a prissy little wimp. "You actually get better from falling," Holm decreed, readjusting a skewed shin guard. "Your balance improves each time. And your body figures out how to fall and not get hurt."

The latter seems debatable, but Holm escapes the day with all limbs and cartilage intact. While he gets plenty of comments from mountain bikers who wonder how he can negotiate a forest on one wheel, Holm is quick to reverse the situation. "Personally, I couldn't imagine riding the North Shore on two wheels!" he countered. Despite the jagged roots and tricked-out trees, Holm feels at home in the North Shore. In 1998, it was here that word began to spread about a guy wheeling through the forests, beaches, and playgrounds of Vancouver on half of a bicycle.

Todd Fiander, nine-time producer of the famed *North Shore Extreme* mountain bike videos, caught wind of Holm and starred him in the video *North Shore Extreme II.* "I put the scary in scary stuff," said Fiander, known for building impossibly dangerous mountain bike trails. "Some of the drops, man, like 16' high, I had to tell Kris *not* to do stuff." Holm didn't listen. "In some of the film clips you can see my camera shaking," Fiander admitted, "and it's on a tripod!"

Documentary filmmakers soon flocked to Holm, creating some 15 films in the past seven years. More than 30 Indie film festivals, including the prestigious Banff Mountain Film Festival World Tour, ran footage of *One Tired Guy* and *Into the Thunder Dragon*, which featured Holm rolling down everything from snow-packed double-diamond ski slopes to dust-ridden trails in Tibet. Television opportunities began popping up (Holm counts fifty to date), and *Ripley's Believe It or Not* came a-knocking in 2000. They asked Holm to ride whatever was high, sharp, dangerous, and deadly, and for the most part Holm agreed to every feat. After all, this was his chance to spread the word about unicycling, to inspire others to try a new sport, and to show that practice and hard work can pay off. But multimedia loves to milk the hype cow, and Holm was often disappointed at the angle the producers took.

"They set the unicyling footage to screaming music and want to label it as extreme when it's not really like that," Holm lamented. "You're out in the forest, and it is beautiful, quiet, the birds are chirping, and you're with your friends. Then when it's edited, they crunch all the action and extreme stuff together. It looks like I'm a gonzo crazy guy instead of someone who is calculating and working out the ride." Crazy indeed. Holm is quite aware that the media is attracted to him for the death-factor risks he takes.

"TV focuses so much on my riding the edges and ridges of things because it is easy to understand: you fall, you die." But for Holm, the media seems unable to capture the essence of the sport. When Ripley's invited him to ride the edge of a new hotel in Vegas, Holm turned them down. "I said no because I don't want to portray myself as a stunt man—I'm an athlete."

While Holm may be the Thoreau of extreme sport, just happy to be riding through nature, the media is right to make a big deal of his talent. Holm is modest, and his voice quiets down when asked if he's won any major titles. He almost whispers that he won the world championship trials in 1999 and the downhill title in 2002. He established the world side hop record (a combination of high jump and a pop-a-wheelie), hopping 90 cm over a bar in 2002. In 2003, Holm spent time filming documentaries and entered some trials competitions. He had to miss the world championships in 2004 due to teaching a geography class at UBC. In the summer of 2005, Holm won the European Trials Championship.

At 32, Holm seems in the prime of his condition,

despite the fact that the European runner-up was 12 years his junior. The future of unicycling lies in young riders, and Holm sponsors two kids through his company—18-year-old Ryan Atkins and Zack Baldwin (who recently surpassed Holm's side hop record by 5 cm) have joined Kris Holm Unicycles. Holm, however, still remains the godfather of unicycling. Recently, the Discovery Channel nabbed Holm to ride for their adventure-athlete show *Stunt Junkies*. "They want me to ride some ladder-bridges on top of a skyscraper in L.A." Holm said, seemingly unperturbed.

As for training, Holm splits his time between trials (obstacles and skills) and mountain settings in an 80/20 ratio, usually averaging 14 hours per week. Not a lot compared to mainstream pro athletes. "I keep a unicycle in the basement of the building where I work as a geologist and ride every lunch hour," Holm said, also noting that he commutes by bike. While he practices his signature moves, like the pedal grab—where you hook your pedal over an obstacle as an intermediate step to climb onto the obstacle—Holm also prefers just to ride around and have fun. When asked if he needs to train more or less than, say, a cyclist with two wheels, Holm relays the unicycle creed, "Mountain bikers suffer all winter so they can suffer all summer, and unicyclists practice all winter so that in the summer they can look like they're not even trying." Underneath the self-effacing humor, Holm has a solid work ethic. Although he dedicates his free time to free wheeling, the irony of his day job is a stark contrast. With a master's degree in physical geography, Holm works for BGC Engineering as a geomorphologist

"I do risk assessment," Holm explained. "I make sure areas are safe from landslides and other natural disasters."

In other words, the areas Holm declares unsafe for people to live on are exactly the places that he likes to ride. Questionable terrain and natural obstacles are all the more inviting, and Holm has ridden an impressive list of locations: Slovakia, Germany, Mexico, Guatemala, the Himalayas, China, and Hawaii, where he was granted legal access to ride on one-week-old lava in Volcano National Park. "I couldn't touch it, but I could ride on it since my tire didn't melt," Holm explained.

The thought of falling seems not to faze him, whether it is on hot lava or off twenty-story buildings. Whereas most of us look at falling as a 50/50 chance, Holm takes an engineer's approach to calculate the equations of risk, hazard, and consequence. Holm talks about the German TV show *Record Fever*, which, in need of a record in 2004, asked Holm to ride along the railing of a 200'-tall bridge in Hawaii. Although the railing was 1' wide, which is "easy riding" for Holm, there were embedded reflector bumps every 10'. Not wanting to slip and fall to his impending death, Holm rationalized the situation. First, he envisioned the bridge being just a few feet off the ground. With this new visualization, he could better assess the reflector bumps and determined it would be best to ride around them, not over them. Piece of cake, really. And while most athletes feel the need to psyche themselves up for performance, Holm focuses on psyching himself down. When perched on top of a bridge, mountain, or swing set, Holm takes a moment to steady his nerves. "I have a little thing I do when I'm high off the ground. I stop, take a deep breath, roll my eyes around, and get into a good zone. I let everything else go. Then I go. Once you're riding, you're just riding. You don't think about consequences."

But of course, there are consequences. Rocks, trees, reflector bumps—Holm is no stranger to falling. Miraculously, the guy has never broken a bone. Bumps and bruises, sprains and stitches prevail, but somehow he has eluded true physical harm. Considering the logistics of a unicycle, it is a wonder Holm is still anatomically intact. Falls appear to threaten Holm with instant eunich-hood, though he swears that most of the impact is felt in the feet, not the crotch.

"On a unicycle, there is no frame. It'll fall away from you. It's so much worse to fall on a bicycle," Holm winced, handing me the unicycle. "You try." After seeing Holm bound off rocks and fly down mountains on his unicycle, I was certain that pedaling a couple feet would be an easy task. We're at a nearby park, and the flat walking path hardly seems threatening. On land, my balance is good, my core muscles relatively stable. Couldn't be that hard to pedal a couple of feet.

Multiple shin bruises and face plants later, I was unable to even sit on the damn thing without holding on to the shoulders of both Kris and his wife, Shannon, in a death grip. Pedaling was out of the question. Perhaps I got a quarter-revolution around before each unwilling dismount, but an eighth-revolution is probably more accurate. But Holm promises victory if I stick with it.

"Anything that is worthwhile takes time and effort," Holm promised, adding, "There is no one out there that can't ride a unicycle." He doesn't make eye contact with me as he says this. I give the unicycle back. Nearby, a man walking his dog stops and watches Holm take off down the path. "Where's your other wheel, man?" he called after him. Holm smiles but just keeps riding.

SWING FOR THE FENCES
January 2011, espnW

From espnW—On January 8, 2011, a 22-year-old gunman carried out an assassination attempt of Congresswoman Gabrielle Giffords. He shot 19 people, six of them fatally, outside a Safeway supermarket in Tucson, Arizona. Nine-year-old athlete Christina Taylor Green was among the victims.

As a female athlete and a resident of Tucson, Arizona, the tragedy of the massacre that took place on January 8, 2011, hit close to home in many aspects beyond geography. Tucson likes to pretend it's a big city, but those of us who live here know the truth. We're a guppy of a metropolis, and we like it that way. We're a small yet sprawling town of involved citizens, often interconnected to other residents by just one degree of separation. Or fewer. Six days before that fateful Saturday, I was called to jury duty under the Hon. John Roll, the federal judge killed in the shooting. His demeanor removed any sense of unease or tension from the courtroom trial, and he seemed to be a kind and caring man. Concurrently, I taught journalism classes at Pima Community College, where the gunman attended school. Unlike that troubled soul, my students were thoughtful, diligent, and eager to learn. I was on Congresswoman Gabrielle Giffords' e-mail Listserv, through which she regularly asked her constituents how she can make our city

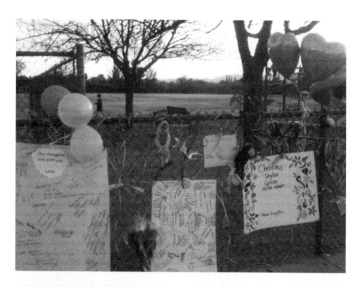

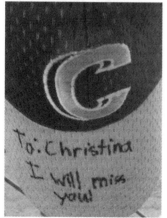

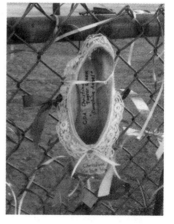

(top) A sign from Christina Taylor Green's Little League team, the Pirates, is a part of a small makeshift shrine at Mesa Verde Elementary School.

(left) The Pirates hung a baseball cap commemorating their fallen teammate.

(right) Christina was a dancer as well as a baseball player. She was enrolled in a class at the Creative Dance Arts academy in Tucson. Many of the dancers signed a decorated toe shoe that is hanging at her elementary school.

better. Her concern and love for Tucson is evident; it transcends partisan lines.

And then there is Christina Taylor Green, the youngest victim in the shooting, a nine-year-old child with whom I've never crossed paths yet to whom I feel a deep connection. This little girl was an athlete, and the bond between female athletes is a quiet, connective thread of respect that ties all its participants together. When I learned Christina was both a dancer and a baseball player, I saw in her a shadow of myself as a young athlete (and, frankly, as an older one). I'm currently an elite cyclist, though I never would have gotten to this level if my love of sports hadn't taken root in childhood, right around Christina's age. Her smile in her Little League team photo portrays the soul of an athlete—here was a little girl who simply loved to play.

According to her coaches at the Canyon del Oro Little League organization, Christina was not just a participant. She was the only girl on her team. She was a baseball enthusiast, a leader on the field and off, and a competitor who held her own against the physicality that comes with playing in a boys' club. She was also born into the game, the daughter of Los Angeles Dodgers scout John Green and the granddaughter of Dallas Green, who managed the 1980 Philadelphia Phillies to the World Series title.

"What Christina exemplified in the baseball arena were the core characteristics we all hope our players will gain from Little League Baseball: character, courage, and loyalty," read a statement by the Canyon Del Oro Little League.

Christina's father coached her Little League team, and that of her 11-year-old brother, Dallas. But it was another coach of Christina's team, the Pirates, who, through the

Canyon Del Oro Little League website, shared a memory of Christina's tenacity as an athlete.

"Christina was not short on courage," her coach wrote. "She played in a baseball league with boys who were strong and fast, but she never once was fazed about being the only girl on the team in 2010. Nor did a hard-hit ball or a whizzing fastball intimidate her. She had the courage to play every position on the field.

"In one particular game, Christina was having a quality at-bat, seeing the ball well and fouling several balls off. After six or seven pitches, the pitcher accidentally let a fastball go that plunked her pretty good. After picking herself up and dusting herself off, Christina was given the choice to take first base or to finish her at-bat, based on loose instructional league rules. With a slight grimace on her face, but without hesitation, she replied, 'I want to hit.' And hit she did. Her tenacious spirit was pumped up, and she drove a hard-hit ball on the next pitch. Courage was just part of who she was."

As is the case with most exceptional athletes, a life in balance was the key to Christina's happiness. "She was so engaged in everything," her coach wrote. "She was always giving her best and excelling, but she was still capable of being a little girl…wanting to play for the sake of play, climbing the mesquite tree at the park with the rest of the team after practice while parents and coaches talked, laughing at silly jokes…she was a rock star in so many ways, but also a beautiful little girl."

On that fateful Saturday morning in January, at the time the tragedy was unfolding on the northwest side of Tucson, I was with a small herd of elite cyclists on a training ride we call "The Shootout." The name is a reference to the tough old ways of the Wild West, as well as an accurate portrayal of how hard the training ride feels, physically. Once the group rolls out to the outskirts of Tucson, it is every man for himself, as the pace revs up to a most incredibly challenging speed. We lose cyclists along the way, as the pace increases and many drop back from the bunch, having spent all their physical bullets of exertion. I hold on for as long as I can through the 60-mile test across the rural landscape of southwest Tucson.

On Saturday, I was one of two or three women out of 120 total cyclists who show up on The Shootout. The male cyclists accept my presence, and I'm grateful for how far we've come in society. Thirty or 40 years ago, this might not have been the case. I'm grateful to the Billie Jean Kings, the Kathrine Switzers, the "Tubby" Johnstons (the first woman to play Little League back in the 1950s), and the Title IX-ers who helped pave the way for the acceptance of female athletes in sports once dominated by men. I often wondered what it was like for kids in the current generation coming up through the sports world, and whether they felt the prejudices of the past.

As it turns out, girls like Christina Taylor Green are a new generation of ambassadors in sport. They not only participate in sports with withering boundaries of gender bias (like baseball), but they're setting newer, bigger goals. In 2010, the registered number of Little League participants in America was 2.7 million children under the age of 18. Of that total, 1,617,000 were between the ages of five and nine. And 163,000 were little girls like Christina Taylor Green, who played mostly on teams comprised of boys. Shortly before her death, Christina told her father she wanted to be the first woman to play in Major League Baseball. While

Christina was robbed of this dream for herself, there is comfort to be found in the immortality of the athletic spirit. She has helped lay the groundwork for other little girls to carry on her dream. Such is the beauty of being a female athlete. Generation by generation, we shape our sports, our games, and our competition to rise to a new level of excellence.

In her brief nine years, Christina Taylor Green both upheld and continued an athletic legacy, whether she knew it or not. The members of her Little League baseball team are boys who will grow up to believe a girl playing baseball is as normal as a guy playing baseball. Those boys will become men who teach their children the same values. Someday there will be a woman in the majors—it's a question of when, not if—and Christina's dream will come full circle for a different female Little League player.

On the way home from my Saturday slugfest of a cycling workout, a friend pulled out his phone. There was a text message advising everyone to avoid Oracle Road in the northwest part of Tucson. A congresswoman had been shot; several people were dead; chaos reigned. By the time we arrived back at our homes, news of the day's events was all over television. As Christina's story was unfolding, I couldn't help wondering if our paths had ever crossed. I have cycled past her northwest Tucson ballfield hundreds of times. Surely she had seen cyclists pass by the windows of her parents' car en route to Little League practice. Our athletic roads less taken, did they ever intersect?

Despite a nearly 30-year age gap and the fact we've never met, Christina's death hit me hard. We were two athletes going about our lives, with very different sports goals stemming from exactly the same foundation. We were playing for the sake of play and to see if maybe, just maybe, we could make the big leagues of our sport. Though she can no longer chase her dream, she's given me a newfound strength and inspiration to chase mine. And as all female athletes know, inspiration is how we leave our mark on the world.

While the loss of Christina Taylor Green is an unfathomable tragedy for our country and our small city of Tucson, her legacy as an athlete does not have to end with the end of her short life. We can honor her life by encouraging girls to play sports, to get involved in class politics, to volunteer their time, to dream of major league debuts and local dance recitals. And when faced with society's equivalent of wild pitches, we can give these girls the courage to swing for the fences. Just like Christina did.

EPILOGUE

ONE OF THE GREATEST GIFTS of sport is the way it challenges our perception of the world, often pushing our intellectual boundaries as it does our physical ones. While there are always athletes who live solely inside their own perceptions, never fully grasping the incredible yet sometimes subtle facets of their journey, most come to understand that sport has deep connections to societal growth and progress. In the midst of my whirlwind introduction into cycling via ESPN's "So You Wanna Be an Olympian?" column, I had little choice but to grab the reigns of this quest and hold on for dear life as it galloped through two years of the most incredible blur of sport. Yet through the dizzying pace of a wild dream on the loose, I remembered to look around now and then. Questions began to arise, many of them forming the basis of the essays in this book. Above all, one question tugged hardest at both my athlete and journalist heartstrings: "Why is women's pro cycling treated so differently than the men's side of the sport?" At best, present-day women's professional cycling is stuck at the same level of women's professional tennis in the 1970s. For six years, I wondered "Why?"

In 2012, the "Why?" grew much louder. My goal of making it to the pro ranks of cycling was finally realized, and simultaneously I was working as an editor and contributor of espnW. Yet I often became discouraged by sports media's tendency to publish repetitive pieces on big stars of mainstream sports, rarely highlighting the unsung athletes of less publicized sports whose unique and compelling stories begged to be written. Of course, advertising and corporate sponsorships have long held the reins in media and marketing. Not to mention this was the 40th anniversary of Title IX. Not many news sources were willing to take a look at the harsh reality: there's still a long way to go before gender equality in sport.

By that point, the "Why?" was deafening. If print and web media were not heeding my personal call of taking women's cycling up a notch, I wondered if visual media might do the trick. I questioned whether any other female pro cyclists might talk to me on camera about their obstacles, their ambition, and their unconditional love for a sport that was often thankless, cruel, and unresponsive to change. What is the true joy of cycling, I wanted to know, and how do we fix the wrongs? But cycling is still a selective sport—Olympic decisions and pro team selections are not earned automatically in many countries, as committees often choose athletes for these coveted spots—would the women talk to me, or not want to rock the political boat? That question alone fueled my curiosity and sent my wondering into overdrive.

So I brought a $99 flip camera to my races and started talking to my fellow competitors. Their stories, thoughts, and opinions were plentiful, rich, and honest. Not only were they willing to talk, they often ran out my camera battery. In spring of 2012, I gathered up enough courage to say the words out loud: "I am going to make a documentary." Without much else to go on, I knew only that I'd need three things—a crash-course education in documentaries, a giant leap of faith, and a professional cameraman with equipment valued beyond $99.

EPILOGUE

For the next two years, I embarked on a new quest. Navigating the new road of filmmaking proved a fascinating journey (largely without road signs) of finding my way through the dead ends, u-turns, and roundabouts of life both with and without a camera. As the film occupied one aspect of my life, so too did job changes, activist groups, family life, and the stark realization that being on a pro cycling team proved a very different reality than the one I'd naively envisioned. I kept a journal through it all—from the film to the racing to the formation of a Tour de France for women—knowing a single essay would not be possible; this would need to be a full memoir someday. I'm at work on the manuscript now, as the story continues to unfold and my film, *Half The Road: The Passion Pitfalls and Power of Women's Professional Cycling*, makes its debut in 2014. With substantial nerves, utmost hope, and childlike anticipation, I can only wonder where this road will lead.

While most books finish with a certain measure of closure, this essay collection of the road less taken is meant to do the opposite. New roads form where old ones end. The big secret behind choosing a road less taken is that the road doesn't actually lead anywhere. It leads *everywhere*. To go off the grid of normal expectations is itself a lifestyle choice, and one unchartered path ultimately leads to the next and then the next…until suddenly we're forty or sixty or eighty years old and we pause and look around…and we can't always remember exactly how we got here, but here we are, and we're very glad indeed. Somewhere along the way we find our niche. Somewhere along the way the road becomes clear. Somewhere along the way we realize we were never supposed to write down our 10-year plan for the future but rather live a life that could fill up a book about the past 10 years. So that's the road I'll head down next, as soon as it presents itself.

In the meantime, keep tabs on my next adventure through KathrynBertine.com, HalfTheRoad.com, @kathrynbertine, and @halftheroad.

Thank you so much for reading.

—K.B.

ACKNOWLEDGMENTS

THIS ESSAY COLLECTION spans the first seven years of my life in cycling, in which there have been innumerable people who have shaped my experiences. Let's start with Bil Johnson; thank you for posing the original 10-year question and for teaching me that questions are life's greatest gift.

Years ago, Lindsay Berra opened the door to ESPN for me, ultimately leading to the right paths and people who kickstarted my cycling career. Thank you, Lindsay, for the wonderful, heartfelt foreword. Likewise, espnW and *Velo News* kept the literary flow going.

In Belgium, Els Van Schoubroek and Wilfried Nolmans took me in as I floundered my way through the brutal and beautiful experience of European racing.

My original St. Kitts and Nevis cycling family members—Winston Crooke, Greg Phillip, Reggie Douglas, and James Weekes—continue to be my brothers in sport.

John Profaci of Colavita gave me my start in pro cycling, but before Colavita came Trisports, Specialized, Gaverzicht Matexi, and countless guest riding opportunities throughout the world that buoyed my dreams of striving for the Olympics, a pro cycling career, and my ravenous need for life experiences. Thanks, too, to all of the sponsors and race directors who support women's cycling.

Enormous thanks my agent, Andrew Blauner, for believing in my words and making this book happen.

Utmost gratitude to Tom Bast, Karen O'Brien, and the good folks at Triumph Books for championing female athlete/authors along the proverbial (and literal) Road Less Taken.

My parents—thanks for inspiring me in vastly different ways. (Keep on "cheatin'," Dad.)

Pete, Kasia, and Alex—thanks for taking me in on a moment's notice and bolstering the dreams and goals.

And to George Varhola, who surely had no idea life with me would be quite this nuts but came along for the ride anyway. Thanks for the unwavering love, support, and for always cleaning my bike chain. All roads lead home to you.

To the women of pro cycling and all those who are trying to get there—you are the soul of this journey, thank you for sharing the road with me. My couch is yours, my fridge is always open, and the pump's in the garage. Help yourself.

SOURCES

FILM
Pee-wee's Big Adventure (1985)

MAGAZINES
Out Sports (Outsports.com) – Kye Allums
Bicycling (bicyclingmag.com)

NEWSPAPERS
The Arizona Daily Star (from azstarnet digital archives)

NEWS SERVICES
The Associated Press – "NCAA adopts transgender athlete policy"
Wikipedia – Gender verification in sports

WEBSITES
www.uci.ch
www.espn.com
www.espnw.com
www.si.com
www.womenscyclingassociation.com
www.cyclingtips.com.au
www.velonews.com
www.cyclingnews.com
www.europigeons.nl
www.colavita.com
www.abae.co.uk

ABOUT THE AUTHOR

KATHRYN BERTINE IS A PROFESSIONAL ATHLETE, author, activist, and documentary filmmaker. She is the 2013 Caribbean Time Trial Champion and three-time national champion of St. Kitts and Nevis (SKN). She raced for Team Colavita/Fine Cooking in 2012 and 2013, and she currently races for the St. Kitts and Nevis National Team. She has garnered one top 10 and six top 20 UCI finishes, and has competed at six world championships. Bertine holds a BA from Colgate University and an MFA from the University of Arizona. A native of Bronxville, New York, she now lives and trains in Tucson, Arizona.

Athletics have been a constant in Bertine's life since childhood. She is a former Division I rower for Colgate University, a pro figure skater, and pro triathlete — all of which eventually led to the beginning of her road cycling career in 2007. Off the bike, she is a journalist and author of two sports memoirs, *All The Sundays Yet to Come* (Little Brown) and *As Good As Gold* (ESPN Books). She wrote the *So You Wanna Be an Olympian?* column for ESPN and the *Riding with the Pros* column for espnW, where she also worked as senior editor in 2011. As an advocate for equality in women's sports, Bertine started the movement of Le Tour Entier with fellow athletes Emma Pooley, Marianne Vos, and Chrissie Wellington in an effort to bring parity to women's professional road cycling, starting with the Tour de France. Her film, *Half the Road: The Passion, Pitfalls, and Power of Women's Professional Cycling*, is her first documentary.

You can follow her on Twitter at @kathrynbertine and @ halftheroad and @letourentier and at www.kathrynbertine. com & www.halftheroad.com.